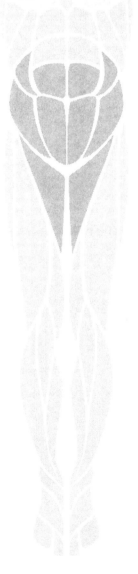

D0937770

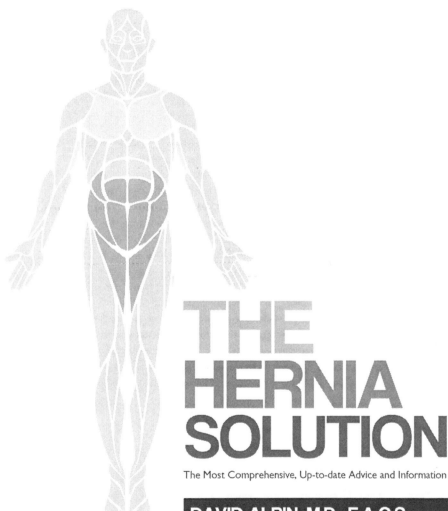

THE
HERNIA
SOLUTION

The Most Comprehensive, Up-to-date Advice and Information

DAVID ALBIN, M.D., F.A.C.S.

Mill City Press, Inc.
212 3rd Avenue North, Suite 290
Minneapolis, MN 55401
612.455.2294
www.millcitypublishing.com

MEDICAL DISCLAIMER

The contents of this book are construed to provide medical information to the general population at large. Each patient is uniquely
different. Therefore, this book should be referred to as a reference
guide. It is not designed to treat or replace the need for a medical
physician. I highly recommend that patients always seek medical
treatment from their personal physician.

DUPLICATED INFORMATION

This book is written as a reference guide that readers can refer
back to when necessary; and as such, each chapter is written as
a stand-alone, containing all of the information needed to fully
understand the concepts under the particular title or subheading.
Some readers may prefer not to read the entire book and will
only be interested in the chapter(s) that apply to their particular medical issue. Thus, each chapter is comprehensive and will
include some duplication of information.

ISBN-13: 978-1-937600-04-4
LCCN: 2011937565

Editor Cliff Carle
Illustrations by John Wu
Book Design by Jenni Wheeler

Printed in the United States of America

FOREWORD

by

Mark Allen

Ironman Triathlon World Champion

I have known Dr. David Albin for several years, having been his coach at several of my triathlon training camps he attended. He is an accomplished surgeon who became a triathlete later in life. As his coach, I can assure you that the heart, determination, and need for excellence he exhibits in his athletic endeavors are also found in the everyday treatment of his patients. As a doctor, he continually strives to better his surgical techniques for the good of his patients, much the same way as an athlete strives to better his performance.

He is dedicated to triathlons and has completed five Ironman races, in addition to many Half Ironman, Olympic, and sprint distance races. Dr. Albin has dedicated his professional life to the treatment and prevention of hernias. Many of his patients are athletes; some are at the professional level.

Just as anyone can get a hernia by simply performing their daily job requirements, or through their daily exercise regime; anyone can sustain the same injuries as a pro athlete while playing "weekend" sports such as basketball, tennis, softball, running, swimming, etc. Hernia injury knows no prejudice; it doesn't discriminate between young or old, male or female, highly active or "weekend warrior". But the knowledge and tools for both prevention and treatment are contained in the book you have in your hands.

Dr. David Albin's book is an excellent resource for anyone who even *thinks* they might have a hernia, or knows of someone who does, and wants to know what steps to take to first fix the hernia and then prevent the hernia from happening again. In *The Hernia Solution*, Dr. Albin answers practically every question you could think of about how the different types of hernias occur, and the essential steps to a fast recovery.

The book also covers sports hernias. Dr. Albin details in-depth rehabilitation programs, broken down by each sport, to help athletes return to their game in top physical condition.

Because Dr. Albin, like myself, has a passionate commitment to excellence in all his endeavors, it is my pleasure to endorse his book, *The Hernia Solution*.

Mark Allen is the six-time Ironman Triathlon World Champion, one of the most difficult one-day sporting events in the world. He graduated from U.C. San Diego, where he was an All-American swimmer, with a degree in biology. He was named Triathlete of the Year six times by *Triathlete Magazine*; and in 1997 *Outside Magazine* tabbed him "The World's Fittest Man". Mark Allen was inducted into the Ironman Triathlon Hall of Fame in 1997. He developed the company Markallenonline.com, renowned for coaching triathletes worldwide, including numerous world champion triathletes. He is also the co-author with Brant Secunda of the award winning book *Fit Soul, Fit Body: 9 Keys to a Healthier, Happier You.*

TABLE OF CONTENTS

INTRODUCTION

FACT: *Hernias affect over 5 million men and women each year.*

Do you suspect that you or a loved one has a hernia?

How dangerous is it?

Should you have an operation now?

What's the worst that could happen if you wait?

What if the operation is not done right and your hernia recurs?

After more than 8000 hernia repairs, Doctor David Albin has developed the new "Albin Technique," integrating several well established procedures with personal variations of his own into a revolutionary method of hernia repair. The result is an operation that combines the best of all tension-free hernia options. Every person in need of hernia surgery should seriously consider requesting this technique. In the year since its discovery, 500+ hernia patients have been treated with the *Albin Technique*. They reported less pain, and returned to work and recreational activities much sooner than the norm. Imagine getting back to the gym, biking, or running only one week after hernia repair surgery! *And most important, not a single hernia has reoccurred in Albin Technique patients.*

As you read *Hernia Solution*, Doctor Albin, the Hernia Specialist, will put your mind at ease with the latest information and a rundown of the most cutting-edge surgical techniques available to help you decide what is best for you. Plus you'll find invaluable post-op care that will reduce pain while getting you back to work and your favorite sport ASAP!

You will have the best surgical results if your operation is performed by a hernia specialist. Determining who the right one for your particular problem is may be difficult. But, armed with the information in this book, you will have an edge.

For many years it was generally accepted that *all* hernias needed surgery. Doctors have recently discovered there are certain types of hernias that may not require immediate attention. This book will help inform you when hernia surgery is absolutely necessary, when you can wait, and when you may not need surgery at all.

It is important you are aware that there are several techniques for repairing hernias. The latest technique that is getting lots of media hype is known as laparoscopic hernia repair. It is the costliest method of hernia repair. Unfortunately, what they sometimes don't tell you is that it can have some serious drawbacks. With the latest information as your guide, *Hernia Solution* will assist in making sure you aren't talked into choosing the wrong operation.

Ladies, are you thinking about getting pregnant, but you're concerned about your umbilical hernia? This book will help you decide which to do first; pregnancy or hernia repair surgery.

Are you an athlete with groin area pain? Doctor Albin is an avid athlete and also specializes in treating sports hernias. He understands the importance of returning to a competitive level of fitness at peak performance. There are multiple tests available when the diagnosis of a hernia is in doubt. The latest protocol will help select the right treatment for you if surgery is deemed necessary. And if your surgeon uses the *Albin Technique* he or she will be able to get you back to your game more quickly.

PREFACE

I, David Albin, am certified by the American Board of General Surgery; I'm a fellow of the American College of Surgeons; and a hernia specialist with over ten years of hands-on experience performing up to 25 operations per week.

This book is a compilation of important facts, findings, and questions that have arisen during my interviewing, diagnosing, and treatment of patients. I felt compelled to write this book because with patient after patient, I kept seeing a need for someone like myself to dispel many of the gross misunderstandings that people have regarding hernias and hernia surgery. It troubles me so see patients who have put off hernia surgery for several years. They've ignored the hernia as if it is "no big deal," while continuing to stoically suffer the aggravation and dull pain.

Unfortunately for some people, while waiting and waiting to undergo what would normally be a minor surgery, their small hernia becomes a larger one resulting in a more difficult operation. Some patients develop serious and even life threatening complications. Often this could have been easily avoided if they had just been better informed.

The most frequent comment that I receive when patients see me for a follow-up exam one week after surgery is, "I should have never waited this long for surgery!"

Other comments are:

"I cannot believe how easy it was to go through the operation."

"I only needed a couple of pain pills."

"I was able to return to work and the gym just one week after surgery."

Some patients do not want to admit that they have a hernia because it is too close to their reproductive organs. They fear that hernia surgery will cause them to lose their sex drive, or even their reproductive ability. None of these sexual myths are true, and you will learn why in this book.

Many women believe that hernias only affect men. The fact is, *no one* is immune from developing a hernia. For the largest percentage of hernias, the only treatment available is surgery. While all surgeries have a risk factor, a hernia operation is one of the safest surgeries you can have—when performed by an *experienced* surgeon—and yet, too often it is indefinitely postponed. Sometimes it's the attitude "I've lived with a hernia this long, what's a few more months—or years?" that prevents them from taking action. And others believe if they ignore their hernia it will eventually go away by itself. Well, I am here to dispel the myths and get you to the truth about hernias

This book was written for everyone. Hernias will affect 10 percent of the general population at some point in their lifetime. Even fully knowing the preventative measures, and always taking the utmost possible care; it even happened to ME! That's right; I developed an inguinal hernia while training for a triathlon race, as you will read in this book.

If it should happen to you or someone you care about, let this book be your guide to quell your fears and bring you peace of mind.

It is my intention that after reading *Hernia Solution*, you will have a complete understanding and be able to make a fully informed decision on how to best treat your particular hernia. But in all circumstances, I highly recommend that you consult with a qualified physician to verify your conclusions.

CHAPTER ONE

FAQs

Frequently Asked Questions

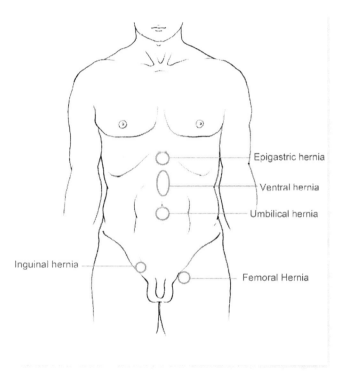

Types of hernias

In my practice as a hernia specialist, patients frequently approach me with their concerns regarding hernias. I have placed these questions in the beginning of the book. Many patients ask the same questions. I answer these questions over and over again. They are concerned regarding their own health, or the health of a loved one. And many times there is only one question that they feel they needed answering before they decide to have hernia surgery. As an example, when patients are diagnosed with a hernia they all want to know: *Is surgery absolutely necessary?*

Over the past several months while I was preparing this book I wrote down the most commonly asked questions. Not all patients need to find out everything there is to know about hernias. They only want their particular questions answered. Once they have the answer they feel they can proceed with certainty. I've also placed these questions and their answers on my Internet site: *www.herniaonline.com*. It is lengthy but quite comprehensive.

My hope is that in this chapter I will answer *your* question and thus help you to make an informed decision. However, the following chapters will go into greater detail for those who wish to have a more in-depth explanation. [NOTE: *Some questions slightly overlap. Thus, certain information will be repeated in order for me to adequately answer each one.*]

What is the difference between a hernia specialist and a general surgeon?

Hernia surgeons are super specialists, and in most cases are board certified general surgeons. They are considered hernia specialists because they limit the majority of their practice to patients who have hernias. Although most general surgeons have the ability to perform hernia surgery within the scope of their practice, they often don't have the same experience associated with hernia surgeons who limit their practice to hernias.

The average general surgeon may perform 25 to 50 hernia surgeries per year, as compared to a hernia surgeon who performs several hundred hernia surgeries annually. Hernia surgeons are skilled, experienced, and have perfected their technique of hernia surgery and the after care of their patients. Although there are general surgeons who can perform excellent hernia surgery, finding them may be difficult.

It is unfortunate that in my hernia practice I see patients who have had surgery preformed by less skilled general surgeons and have developed problems after surgery that I then have to fix. Most general surgeons wisely refer their most difficult hernias to the hernia specialists.

I perform up to 25 hernia operations each week. My patients experience less postoperative pain and are able to return to work sooner than the norm. They are also able to work out and resume recreational activities sooner than the norm.

What is a hernia?

A hernia is a small sac that protrudes through the muscles of the abdominal wall and contains some of the contents of the abdominal cavity, mainly the intestines or fatty tissue. The hernia sac itself is made of the covering layer of the abdominal cavity or the peritoneum (a thin membrane covering the intestinal cavity).

How does a hernia develop?

As the outer layers of the abdominal wall weaken they begin to bulge and actually rip causing internal organs and tissue to push through the tear creating a bulge, which is known as a hernia.

The most common activities that would cause the abdominal wall to weaken are strenuous activities such as heavy lifting, pushing, or pulling. A contributing factor may be a congenital weakness in the muscles which explains why these activities do not affect everyone the same way.

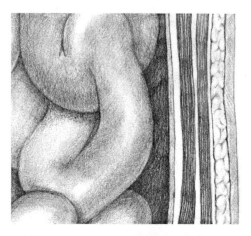

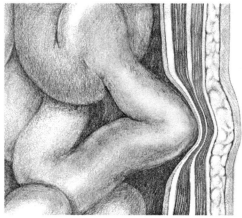

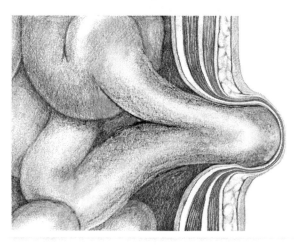

Stages in the development of a hernia: Normal abdominal wall above. Weakened abdominal wall in the middle. Ruptured abdominal wall with bulging intestines below.

The causes of abdominal wall hernias are similar independent of their location. Straining can result in a hernia. The hernia most often occurs in the weakest location in the abdominal wall, which is the inguinal region. The second weakest spot is the umbilical region, and this is also the second most common location for a hernia to develop.

There is not always a defined reason why hernias develop in less common sites resulting in the ventral or epigastric hernias. There may be a congenital weakness in these areas. Some ventral hernias develop in obese patients as a result of constant pressure from within their abdominal cavity caused by excessive fatty tissue on their muscles. Some epigastric or ventral hernias develop on the abdominal wall due to enlarged muscular blood vessels that perforate and weaken the abdominal wall.

I have a bulge in my abdomen, is that a hernia?

An abdominal bulge in the area of the upper or lower abdomen, or the navel, that can be compressed or feels squishy is typically a hernia. The bulge is present in an abnormal location. Normal bulges are that of fat or muscle. Example: Working out at the gym and getting a large muscle or "working out" at the dinner table and getting fatty bulges.

If there is any question or concern—and especially if there is a feeling of discomfort or pain in the area of this bulge, a qualified physician should be consulted to provide you with an accurate diagnosis.

Are hernias painful?

Not all hernias are painful. The law of thirds applies. Approximately one third of my patients with a hernia complain of a bulge without pain.

Approximately one third of my patients have a bulge that is either painful to varying degrees, or simply annoying. In other words, the majority of patients simply complain of an unsightly bulge. Usually the hernia feels *funny* like a squishy feeling, or there's an uncomfortable feeling periodically, or throughout the day. Pain is present in some instances, however it is uncommon except in the acute phase.

The final third of my patients have found that they have an asymptomatic or inconsequential hernia that they did not know about. These hernias were diagnosed at the time of physical examinations by their family physicians. During a routine examination, and to the surprise of the patient, they were told that they have a hernia.

Why is a hernia painful?

In the acute phase, the hernia may be painful when the surrounding muscles tear or rupture. This is similar to what is seen in an acute muscular injury. The torn muscles become very sensitive due to stretching, swelling, and engorgement with blood as you may expect in a common bruise. The nerves in the region of the injury become sensitive to pain.

An inguinal or a groin hernia can cause groin pain. The reason the hernia is painful is due to the hernia sac and its contents being *squashed* as it pushes through the muscles in the inguinal canal, which is the groin region. The hernia compresses the nerves going to the genitalia, or it may actually impede the circulation to the testicles causing pain in the genital region. At times when the hernia contains intra abdominal contents such as the intestines, it is compressed by the abdominal muscles, which pinch the intestines or abdominal contents causing pain.

Can a woman get a hernia in the groin area?

Contrary to popular belief, women can also get groin hernias. They experience the same symptoms as men do when this occurs. Hernias are 85 percent more common in men than in females. This is primarily because men tend to perform more strenuous work. However, groin hernias are becoming more prevalent in women who are, for example, fire fighters, construction workers, paramedics, police officers, soldiers, etc.

What are the locations a hernia can develop?

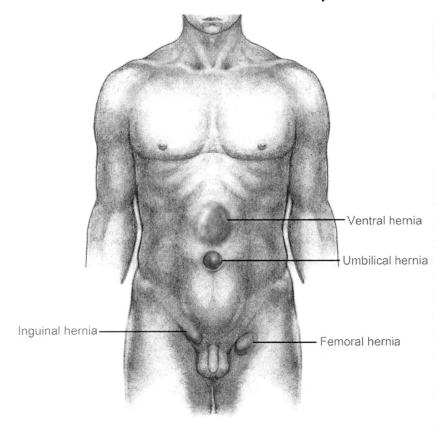

Location of common hernias

Although the groin area is the most common site for a hernia, an abdominal hernia can occur at any place in the abdominal cavity.

Inguinal or groin hernias develop in the inguinal regions. This is the lower portion of the abdomen near the genital region and just above the thigh. Inguinal hernias begin in the groin area and as they enlarge they can either travel to the scrotum (in males) or the labia (in females). Femoral hernias occur in the groin just below the skin crease.

The second most common region is the umbilicus or naval (belly button) region. The other locations include multiple locations in the abdominal wall. This occurs more commonly in the midline, typically between the umbilicus or belly button and the sternum or chest cavity. These locations are known to be ventral hernias or epigastric hernias. In addition, a ventral hernia can occur in other locations of the abdominal wall on either side of the midline.

After having had an operation on my abdomen I have developed a bulge—can a hernia develop after abdominal surgery?

There is a hernia known as an incisional hernia which occurs in an improperly healed incision. In this instance the abdominal contents are able to push through the improperly closed abdominal wall wound causing a hernia.

Do all hernias require surgery?

In almost all instances a hernia will not go away without surgery. There is no medication to treat a hernia. There is no exercise to treat a hernia. Exercise will strengthen the abdominal wall muscles but that will not make the hernia go away.

The abdominal cavity contains the abdominal contents such as the intestines, stomach, liver and other organs. The abdominal wall can be compared to a girdle or a corset. When the abdominal wall tears, a hernia develops. There is a constant positive pressure from the abdominal contents that is placed on the abdominal wall. This mechanical force, maintained by the abdominal contents, keeps the muscles separated. The muscle can heal itself to some extent such as seen in a strained or bruised muscle. Exercise can strengthen the muscles, but cannot repair the damage.

A muscle has two primary attachments. One is called the origin and the other is the insertion. The easiest way to imagine this is by thinking of the muscles of the limbs. When the muscles contract, the joint bends. If one attachment is covered, the joint no longer is able to bend. Although the muscle can heal itself, it cannot reattach itself. The muscle cannot completely regenerate itself, as an amputee cannot regenerate a limb. Therefore, hernias need surgery to close the gap between either sides of the muscle tear. That is why there is no medicine or exercise that will make a hernia go away.

One exception is infantile hernias that develop during pregnancy, which may heal without surgery. Infantile umbilical hernias will heal by themselves if the abdominal wall completes its development, usually by age five. After age five it's unlikely that infantile hernias will close.

Another exception is in regard to pregnant women. During the course of pregnancy as the abdominal wall enlarges, at times a hernia will develop in the umbilical region which will spontaneously close after delivery within the first couple of months.

Once a hernia has been repaired, what is the chance of developing another hernia?

In general, patients with one hernia are as unlikely to develop a second hernia as those patients who've never had a hernia. The abdominal wall should regain its original strength by virtue of the hernia repair. However, the patients who frequently develop hernias do so by improper lifting. If they are able to correct their lifting techniques it is unlikely that another hernia will develop.

Improper lifting can result in a hernia because the amount of force placed on the muscle can tear the muscle tissue in a manner similar to the way continually pulling a rubber band can make it snap. By using proper lifting techniques, the force of the strenuous activity is distributed among several muscles, primarily the larger muscles. To avoid placing too much stress on the abdominal muscles, it is better to lift using your legs and maintaining good posture, rather than using your back and abdominal muscles.

After hernia surgery will I be able to resume my regular activities?

Patients frequently ask me if, after surgery, they will be able to return to their regular activities without fear of developing another hernia. Some of the laborers want to know if they will need a permanent restriction on lifting. Weightlifters want to know if they need to give up their sport. This is a valid question because prior to the development of hernia mesh, hernias were repaired under tension using several sutures. After this type of an operation, the patients were frequently told that they should not lift over forty pounds.

With the development of the tension-free mesh technique such as the methods that I perform, patients can return to lifting without fear of developing a recurrent hernia. This is because the repair is done without tension and the material used in the mesh is permanent. Many of the materials used are several times stronger than the pre-injury strength of the muscles.

Imagine tearing your trousers in the crotch. The finest Italian tailor has the ability to repair the tear with such exactness that that the tear is practically invisible. It may look good, but when you sit down the pants will feel tight and may re-tear in the same spot. On the other hand, if the tear were to be repaired loosely with a large strong patch, it is unlikely that it would tear a second time. The tension-free mesh hernia repair acts in the same way.

If I have a groin hernia repaired on my right side, does my left side have a chance of tearing from the same activity?

Yes. The repaired side, using the tension-free mesh technique, is stronger than the normal abdominal wall muscles. If a patient has had the right side repaired and they perform a similar activity that caused the first hernia, they are more likely not to develop a recurrent hernia, rather a new hernia on the left side. That is why it is better that we learn from our mistakes and avoid improper lifting and straining.

Can a hernia lead to or cause a urological dysfunction?

Nothing in medicine is absolute. But as a rule, a hernia will not cause a urological dysfunction. Some patients are reluctant to undergo hernia surgery because they fear that they will lose their manhood, or that they will not be able to perform sexually. Hernia surgery will not cause this to occur. Others feel that they run the risk of sterilization by losing a testicle. It is unlikely that hernia surgery will result in the removal of a testicle.

Will I be able to resume regular sexual activity after hernia surgery?

Hernia surgery will not affect sexual activity; however some patients may have a diminished motivation if they experience genital pain after surgery.

Patients can resume sexual activity after hernia surgery as soon as they become comfortable. Most patients need a week of abstinence due to discomfort. Some will require more and others less time for resuming sexual activity. I tell my patients that they can resume sexual activity a day or two after after surgery if they are very gentle.

Will sexual activity be painful after hernia surgery?

Some patients with a hernia may find sexual activity painful. This commonly occurs with large hernias. Their body may associate sexual activity with pain. This becomes a learned response. After surgery it may take awhile before the body forgets this learned response. Eventually sexual activity will no longer be painful. For the most part, it is unlikely that a properly preformed hernia repair will cause painful sexual activity.

Some painful inguinal hernias have been known to interfere with an erection. The pain is reduced when the erection is reduced. This is a self-defense mechanism. After repairing the hernia, which is the cause of the problem, sexual function should return to normal. Sometimes, following hernia surgery, there is a delay in return to normal erectile function, especially if the problem has been there for some time. Often though, the delay is more psychological than physiological, and is generally due to the fear that was associated when the hernia was present.

After hernia surgery will I have pain?

Patients may experience severe pain for the first couple days after hernia surgery. Mild temporary pain is common after ANY operation. Generally, this mild pain will last for a few weeks then diminish and eventually disappear. But it is not uncommon for mild infrequently occurring pain to last up to a year. Long lasting chronic pain is rare. It affects a very small percentage of hernia patients.

Am I going to be 100% recovered?

I tell the majority of my patients that they will be 95% of their pre-injury state. After any surgery there will be some reminder of the surgery.

Unfortunately, I find many disappointed patients coming to me *after* they have had surgery *elsewhere*. They are still suffering from pain weeks and months after their hernia surgery. Their doctors told them that they would be back to 100 percent shortly after surgery, and they returned to normal activity too soon. It is a misrepresentation if you are told that you will be back to 100 percent directly after surgery. Sadly, some surgeons are afraid that the absolute truth might prevent their patients from having the surgery unless it's an emergency; or that it might scare them away altogether.

I never tell my patients that they will be back to 100 percent without qualification of this answer. No matter what operation that you have, there is always a lingering discomfort reminding you of the operation. I refer to this as the "95 percent rule." Most certainly patients will be able to perform the same activities that they did before surgery. However there will be an occasional cramp or twinge of pain reminding them of their hernia operation. This will last for about a year. After a year they will be at or very near 100 percent recovery.

Will I need hospitalization for hernia surgery?

A typical routine uncomplicated hernia operation can be performed as outpatient surgery, outside of a hospital setting.

At my outpatient surgery center, I perform hernia surgery in about forty minutes. Patients leave the facility another thirty minutes after their operation. You cannot imagine how simple this can be. From the time patients reach the waiting room within less than two hours they are on their way home. There is no need for hospitalization. Hernia surgery is almost always performed as an outpatient. The exception is patients with vary large hernias or complicated medical problems. In these cases hospitalization is required.

How soon after surgery can I return to work?

Returning to work depends on the type of work you do. Patients who work at home or on a computer can usually return to work within a couple of days.

An office worker with a typical desk job is generally able to return to work within a week.

The patient with laborious work that is intermittent where there is occasional lifting of average weights, moderate strenuous activities in the range of 40 pounds, can usually go back to work within two weeks.

The patients who have strenuous work where they are continuously lifting, pushing and pulling throughout the course of the day, will return to regular work within four weeks.

The patients who have very strenuous work where they are continuously lifting, pushing and pulling heavy loads throughout the course of the day will return to regular work within four to six weeks.

When can I resume physical activity after surgery?

Physical activity can usually be resumed within a week after surgery. Patients return to physical activity in moderation with a gradual building up of the activity. It usually takes about a month to return to pre-hernia exercise or activity levels.

Is a hernia surgery dangerous?

In general, hernia surgery is not dangerous, although it is considered a major operation. But as major operations go, this is one of the least invasive.

In my practice I have preformed over 8000 hernia operations. I have never had an immediate postoperative emergency because my patients are all screened for medical problems prior to surgery.

If the patient has a medical problem my team will optimize their health prior to surgery. I have never had a surgical death as a result of my hernia surgery.

I have experienced two unexpected hernia recurrences. They were both successfully repaired. Since then my technique has been modified to prevent their type of recurrence from happening.

We currently average one infection out of two hundred hernia patients. However, obese patient are ten times more likely to develop an infection after hernia surgery than other patients. Several years ago we developed a greater incidence of infections at one hospital. I handled this by personally overseeing the preparation of my surgery patients, and at that hospital we have not had an infection in four years.

Most hernia infections are handled with oral or topical antibiotics. One out of five hundred of my patients require a minor surgery to treat their infection. They have all recovered with no other problems. They return to work after their infection has subsided, which amounts to usually no more than a one week delay.

In my postoperative orders, I state that hernia patients need to go *directly home* after surgery and *rest*. I have an average of one patient every other year go to the hospital after surgery because they feel so good after hernia surgery that they disobey my postoperative orders, and dine in a restaurant immediately after surgery. They often feel dizzy, and one even fainted in the restaurant. Paramedics were called and they returned home after a few hours of observation in the emergency room.

Some hernia patients are at a higher risk due to multiple failed hernia operations, extreme obesity, or steroid usage. I make sure they are informed in advance that they are at high risk for hernia recurrence.

Is there a risk of needing a blood transfusion during hernia surgery?

None of my hernia patients have ever required a blood transfusion either during or after hernia surgery. Hernia surgery is typically bloodless and does not require a blood transfusion. The average blood loss from hernia surgery is less than 5 cc which is the amount of blood contained a small test tube, and is similar to the amount which is withdrawn when your personal physician performs a standard blood test.

What happens if the mesh becomes infected?

Mesh infections are very rare. If an infection does occur it can usually be treated with a course of oral antibiotics lasting one to four weeks depending on the seriousness of the infection. The mesh rarely has to be removed. In my practice I am extremely careful in avoiding mesh infections. Only once in my practice did I have to place a patient of mine on intravenous antibiotics for a mesh infection that occurred as a result of hernia surgery in the hospital. And I have never had to hospitalize a surgery center outpatient of mine for intravenous antibiotics. I have never had to remove an infected mesh from any of my hernia patients.

Do I have to go to sleep for hernia surgery?

No, as a general rule, hernia surgery can be done either under local anesthesia, or local anesthesia with sedation. Large difficult hernias although will require general anesthesia in some cases.

What if the patient has existing medical problems?

Some patients with hernias have pre-existing medical conditions such as diabetes, high blood pressure or heart disease. Although surgery is necessary for these patients, it is advised that they see their regular physician or a specialist so that they will be in their best physical condition prior to surgery. In instances where surgery is risky in patients with medical problems, hernia surgery can usually be safely performed under local anesthesia with sedation.

What is the difference between a reducible and an incarcerated hernia? And what is a strangulated hernia?

Reducible hernias can be pushed back inside the abdomen. Non-reducible (also called incarcerated) hernias cannot be placed back into the abdomen. A strangulated hernia is an incarcerated hernia that has developed an additional complication: The blood supply to the hernia has been cut off and now emergency surgery is required.

Incarcerated hernias should be operated on an urgent basis. If strangulation is present then the patient may not be able to have mesh placed. Strangulated hernias develop severe complications including infections, so mesh is usually not placed. When a strangulated hernia is repaired without mesh the reoccurrence rate is higher than an elective reducible hernia repair. To avoid this complication it is obviously better to have surgery before incarceration or strangulation occurs.

Any reducible hernia can develop into a non-reducible or incarcerated hernia. It can occur anytime. There is no advance notice. There are no warning signs. And there is no ballpark time when this can occur. I advise my patients to have their hernia repaired within six weeks of diagnosis. After this time they are skating on thin ice. When this change in the status of the hernia occurs, surgery is needed on an urgent basis. If they are in a location where medical aid is unavailable their life is at risk. If they are late in getting help, the hernia may become a life-threatening emergency if not immediately resolved.

This is a notice to all hernia patients to seek immediate medical attention whenever you suspect that you might have a hernia.

Who gets hernias?

According to the American Medical Association and the National Center for Health Statistics, estimates are that about five million people in the United States suffer from hernias every year. This is a well-accepted statistic.

Most of these adults develop hernias from sudden or repeated stress or strain in the abdominal muscles. Some hernias may be congenital (from birth).

What types of activities cause hernias?

The types of activities associated with hernias involve an increase in the abdominal pressure as a result of lifting heavy objects, sudden twists or pulls, or muscle strains. Frequent straining with urination, chronic constipation, or chronic coughing can also cause a hernia.

What is the cost of a hernia?

The cost can be divided into medical and non-medical expenses.

The medical expenses include: the surgeon's fee, hospital fees, the anesthesia fees and the laboratory fees.

The non-medical costs may be more expensive as they stem from the loss of productivity as a result of time away from work. However, in some instances, patients are able to use a paid leave of absence for their surgery, for example paid sick leave, or the second or third week of a vacation.

Non-expensive costs that should be considerably factored is lost time off of recreational activity. This involves one's inability to participate in recreation such as sport activities.

Below is an estimate of the cost of a routine single hernia. A complicated, double, or recurring hernia can cost between 50 to 100 percent higher:

	Low	High
Surgeon	$ 1000	$ 2000
* Surgery center	2000	--
* Hospital	--	7000
Anesthesia	200	600
Lab	50	200
Totals	**$ 3250**	**$ 9800**

* Note: Patients will require surgery either at a surgery center or a hospital.

Are larger hernias more expensive?

Yes. As the hernia enlarges, which occurs over time, the expense will increase. Both medical and non-medical expenses will likely increase. If left untreated and complications arise, the expenses can be stifling with the end result of a loss of many months of activity at work and chronic problems as a result of a less than adequate surgical result. Many of these potential expenses can be minimized by early surgical intervention and repair.

Is hernia surgery an emergency?

Hernias that are reducible, although they can be painful, do not require urgent surgery. They can be repaired on an elective basis. A non-reducible hernia is in danger of strangulation and requires emergency surgery.

What happens if I have a double hernia?

I treat double hernias no differently than single hernias. Postoperatively, it is more painful to have two hernias repaired as compared to one hernia. As a rule, the pain and the recovery time for a double hernia is about 50 percent more than a single hernia. For this reason most patients prefer to undergo one hernia operation at a time. Also, when a patient has multiple medical problems I insist on operating on one hernia at a time. A patient with medical problems and two hernias may not tolerate a lengthy operation associated with a double hernia repair. It is safer to stage the operations at separate sittings. One hernia operation is preformed first. The patient is allowed to sufficiently recover prior to performing the second operation. This usually takes about one or two weeks.

Am I more likely to get a hernia on the right side or the left side?

Hernias occur more commonly on the right side. There is no explanation for this.

Will my hernia go away on its own?

No medicine will make a hernia go away. There is no exercise that can be performed to repair a hernia. Physical therapy cannot heal a hernia. A hernia is the result of a defect in the muscles, usually due to a tear. The muscle needs to be surgically repaired. Although a hernia may not enlarge for months or years, if untreated it will never go away on its own. Surgery is the only option to repair a hernia.

That said; let me now lead you through a more in-depth understanding of the hernia…

CHAPTER TWO

Interviewing the Hernia Patient

The Symptoms of a Hernia

Individuals will experience different symptoms depending on the type of hernia as well as the individual's overall health and well-being. In order to properly diagnose a hernia, your doctor will perform a physical exam and review your symptoms to first determine whether or not there is a hernia present.

The symptoms of a hernia are the presence of a bulge in an unexpected location on the abdominal wall that may or may not be painful. Less common symptoms are urinary disturbances associated with frequent urination or urinary infections. This occurs when the hernia contains the urinary bladder. Rare symptoms are constipation, nausea and vomiting. This occurs when the intestines are involved and the hernia is becoming incarcerated.

A Bulge is the Most Common Symptom

The more common symptoms are those of a swelling or a bulge that is underneath the skin. The hernia is a small sac that protrudes through a hole or a defect in muscles of the abdominal wall. The hernia sac may contain some of the contents of the abdominal cavity, mainly the intestines or fatty tissue. The bulge may initially have a squishy feeling when pressed and may even temporarily disappear. This bulge is known to appear while you are standing and disappear while you are lying down, because of gravity. Imagine a glass of water open at the top. The open glass represents the neck of the hernia. Upright the contents remain in the glass but when the glass tips over the contents spill outside. In a similar fashion the hernia contents disappear when you lie down and protrude in a standing or sitting position.

A bulge or a swelling occurs because of a hole or defect in the abdominal wall muscle. When this happens, the abdominal contents, usually fat within the abdominal cavity or even intestinal contents protrude outwards. This bulge or swelling is known as a hernia. The intestinal contents are contained within a sac. The sac, called peritoneum, is also referred to as the hernia sac.

While performing strenuous activities there is an increase in abdominal pressure. Over time, strenuous activities such as lifting, straining or coughing tend to cause an increase in abdominal pressure. Eventually, the muscle fibers give way, tear slightly, and the internal pressure forces a small portion of the peritoneum through the small hole in the abdominal wall. The resulting bulge is the hernia.

Pain Associated with Hernias

Pain is best explained with the rule of thirds. One third of hernia patients have no pain. One third have a discomforting or uncomfortable feeling that is mildly annoying. One third have serious pain. Pain or discomfort occurs in the immediate area of the bulge or throughout the abdomen.

Approximately one third of the patients have a bulge that is not at all painful or discomforting. It is "just there." Some of my patients experience no pain, rather they complain of a "funny feeling," or a bulge in the groin that was not there before. A person who is very physically active, such as an athlete, or a worker who performs arduous labor is more likely to develop a hernia without feeling any pain. But it is unwise to ignore a bulge of any size, even if it is not painful. You should have it examined by a physician regardless.

Approximately one third of hernia patients have either a mildly painful or discomforting bulge. This discomfort is often described as a "funny feeling;" or a feeling that "something is there." That is, a bulge that was not present before, and not noticeable, ongoing pain.

A person who is very physically active, such as an athlete, or a worker who performs arduous labor, may experience only intermittent discomfort. In some instances, during the phase when the abdominal wall is rupturing, resulting in a hernia, patients will complain of an ache similar to a muscle strain, instead of a sharp pain. This is a more typical complaint for patients who are constantly performing strenuous activities. They think muscle strain is a routine part of their daily routines. If they work hard some days they are a little sorer than usual. But it's the specific location of the soreness which may in fact be the hallmark of the development of a hernia.

Annoying or severe pain occurs in approximately the final one third of hernia patients. This pain may intensify as the hernia develops. This is called the acute phase, and is the result of muscle tissue stretching or tearing, and impinging upon the surrounding nerves. When the tissues around the hernia are stretched or torn these tissues, which contain nerve endings, experience a painful response. For these patients, due to the intense discomfort, it is very clear that there is something wrong. The type of intense pain associated with a hernia can be described several ways: a burning pain, a tearing pain, sharp, dull or point pain.

A hernia can also cause a radiating pain which occurs away from the site of the hernia—or a generalized pain, which is a pain throughout the abdominal cavity. A hernia can also cause referred pain (sensations of pain in other areas away from the actual site of the hernia). This is because the irritated nerve travels along the nerve fibers to other regions supplied by the same nerve. For example, patients with a hernia may complain of pain in the testicle or the inner thigh. In this case, the irritated nerve at the site of the hernia has traveled along its path to the testicle or thigh. In some instances the effected nerve may actually travel *back* to the abdomen resulting in pain that starts in the groin and radiates along the flank to the back. This pain is similar to the pain caused by testicular trauma because the nerve to the testicle travels backwards to the abdomen and the back. Thus, referred pain can occur anywhere along the course of the nerve from the site of origin in the groin, to the testicle and thigh, or inwards to the abdomen and back.

The pain that occurs during the hernia development usually subsides in a week or two. If you develop a hernia, even if you no longer experience pain, it is important to remember that the hernia will not go away on its own. Even if the pain has subsided, surgery is the only treatment to correct or undo the hernia.

Severe Pain Symptoms

In severe cases a hernia can cause generalized pain when incarceration or strangulation occurs. The intra abdominal organs such as the intestines become pinched resulting in a diminished blood supply. The diminished blood supply causes an irritation of the nerves supplying the intestines, resulting in intense pain. The pain from a strangulated hernia, which starts as a stomachache, and increases in severity, may result in nausea and vomiting. If untreated, the strangulated intestines may rupture with fatal results if prompt surgery is not performed.

A physician should be immediately consulted to determine the cause of any severe pain. In some instances, the pain, while appearing to be a hernia may actually be due to a non hernia cause. A few common causes of abdominal pain are an appendicitis, cholecystitis, peptic ulcer disease, or an ovarian cyst. These should be ruled out throughout the course of physical examination.

Constipation as a Symptom

Constipation occurs when a portion of the large intestines are within the hernia sac. The stool within the intestine becomes mechanically blocked by the hernia. At times, if the blood flow to the intestine is blocked, the stool will be unable to travel through the intestines. This will result in either constipation or blood in the stool. When this occurs, emergency surgery is necessary.

Nausea and Vomiting

Nausea and vomiting may also occur when a hernia becomes incarcerated or strangulated. The flow of food in the intestines may become blocked by the hernia sac. The backup that results within the intestine may cause nausea or vomiting. The nausea and vomiting occur as a result of a partial or complete blockage of intestine. In addition, loss of appetite may occur. The treatment of an intestinal blockage resulting in nausea and vomiting is considered emergency surgery.

Urinary Symptoms

Urinary disturbances may occur when the bladder is within the hernia sac. In this instance, a portion of the urinary bladder has been trapped by the hernia. The more common urinary disturbances result in frequent urination due to an inability to completely empty the bladder. A common symptom is urinating frequently during the day and several times at night.

When the bladder is chronically trapped within the hernia, a urinary infection may develop. A urinary infection may cause burning urination, urinary frequency, and bloody urination. Additionally, patients with prostate problems are also known to develop hernias. As the prostate enlarges, the patient tends to strain during urination, and the constant straining may result in the formation of a hernia.

Physical Examination:

If a physical examination of the patient by a trained physician reveals an abnormal bulge in the abdominal wall, it is highly likely that a hernia is present. The bulge usually is not exceptionally tender to the touch. In rare instances the bulge has become very tender. A very tender bulge may be present if the hernia is incarcerated or strangulated. The hernia bulge may or may not be reducible depending on whether or not it is incarcerated.

On the other hand, newly developed hernias may be tender due to the

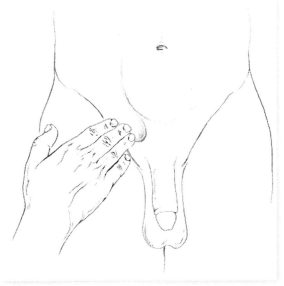

Examination of an inguinal hernia patient.

recent tear in the muscle. In most cases, the bulge is present in the location of the hernia. Hernias may be located anywhere on the abdominal wall. The most common location is the inguinal or groin region. The second most common location is the umbilical region. Ventral hernias occur anyplace on the abdominal wall but are most common in the midline. Incisional hernias occur in previous surgical incisions.

When hernia symptoms occur, but a hernia is not visibly present on physical examination, an X-ray may be necessary to determine if a hernia is actually present. The initial radiological examination usually performed is an abdominal ultrasound. If this exam is unable to definitively determine whether or not a hernia is present, a CT scan or MRI may demonstrate the presence of a hernia. An examination called a "herniaogram," which is less commonly used these days, may identify a hernia. As a last resort, exploratory surgery will definitely determine if a hernia is present.

In addition to performing a hernia exam it is important for your doctor to perform a general health exam. It is essential to auscultate the lungs because patients with a chronic cough are prone to developing a hernia and this should be treated prior to hernia surgery. An abdominal exam is necessary to determine if there is any abdominal tenderness or additional abnormal swellings. A rectal exam should be done to determine if there is blood in the stool or an enlarged prostate. An enlarged prostate can lead to urinary straining and hernia formation. A patient with an enlarged prostate will have urinary symptoms and should be referred to a urologist.

A doctor may ask during a hernia exam:

- How long have you had the hernia?
- How did you develop the hernia?

- What other medical problems do you have?

Dr. Albin asks the following additional questions that other doctors may not think of:

- What type of recreational activities or sports do you perform?
- What is your skill level?
- How much time is left in your season?
- How much time do you spend working out each day?
- To weightlifters: What amount of weight do you lift?
- What activities or work do you intend to do after your surgery?

This allows me to customize a hernia repair to meet their individual needs as well as to determine the timing of their hernia repair.

CHAPTER THREE

Types of Hernias

There are many types of hernias. The more common types of hernias are the inguinal or groin hernias and the umbilical or navel hernias. A less common type is the ventral hernia which can occur in any place of the abdomen. Epigastric hernias occur in the midline below the breast bone. Femoral hernias occur just below the crease of the groin. The more rare types of hernias include incisional hernias, which result in the tissue of a scar. A spigellian hernia presents in the front of the abdomen, below the umbilicus on the right or left side. The obturator hernia is a very rare pelvic hernia. A hiatal hernia is caused by a defect in the diaphragm.

Obturator and hiatal hernias are not considered abdominal wall hernias because they are located internally within the abdominal cavity. Since they are treated by general surgeons and not hernia specialists, they are not covered in this book.

Sports hernias are a type of inguinal hernia that occur primarily in professional-level athletes and will be discussed in a separate chapter.

The Inguinal Hernia

Inguinal hernias are also known as groin hernias. They occur in the region of the groin between the lower abdomen and the thigh. They are the most common adult hernia. They range in size from about one to two inches.

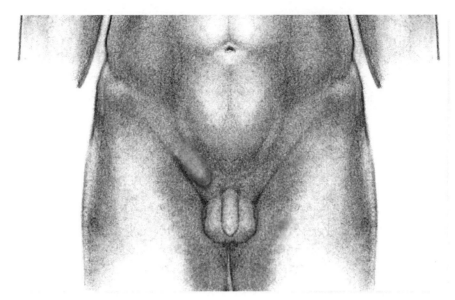

Inguinal hernia.

However, inguinal scrotal hernias which enter the scrotum area tend to be much larger. Inguinal hernias are far more common in men than females. The inguinal hernia occurs as a result of a weakness or a tear in the abdominal wall muscle creating a bulge. The bulge contains a sac of peritoneum, which is also the covering of the intestinal cavity. In addition, the contents of a hernia may contain intestine, fat or omentum (fatty tissue inside the abdominal cavity which covers and protects the intestines).

Inguinal hernias may occur on the right side, the left side, or simultaneously on both sides of the groin. Inguinal hernias typically are the result of strenuous activities. In younger adults and children they may be congenital in origin. Hernias may also be a result of straining during constipation, difficultly with urination, or the presence of chronic coughing.

At times a hernia may be painful. At other times there may be no pain at all—or just mild discomfort. The pain or discomfort you feel is caused by straining the abdominal muscles which causes a pinching in the hernia sac or its contents. The pain may be constant or intermittent, occurring most noticeably with strenuous activities.

The degree of pain will vary from one individual to another. But it is important to know that the absence of pain does not mean that the hernia poses no medical problem. Sooner or later, all inguinal hernias will require surgery to correct. Regardless of how painless they are, they will never go away on their own. There is no such thing as a self-correcting hernia.

The resulting scar following the tension-free mesh repair that I use varies between one to two inches in length depending on the size of the patient. An overweight patient will usually have a larger scar than smaller individuals. A bathing suit will generally cover the scar.

My patients begin a rehab program one day after surgery. I encourage my patients to begin walking the day after their operation. One week after surgery they are already stretching and participating in aerobic exercises. After two weeks, patients will begin using light weights. I have found that an early rehab program enables my patients to have a speedy return to exercise and work. Overall, they feel better sooner.

The Umbilical Hernia

Umbilical hernias occur in the umbilical or navel region, also known as the belly button. As with inguinal hernias, the umbilical hernia is a result of a weakening or tearing of the abdominal wall muscle through which the intestinal contents protrude. They range in size from one to four inches.

Umbilical hernias may be congenital in origin, occurring at birth. The umbilical hernias may also result from strenuous activities or medical factors such as coughing, straining a stool, or difficulty with urination. The umbilical hernia is more prevalent in women due to the abdominal wall stretching that occurs during pregnancy.

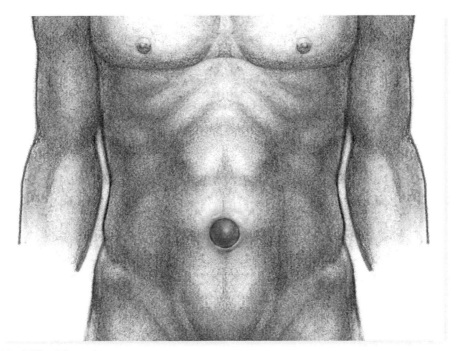

Umbilical hernia

The majority of umbilical hernias will not go away without surgery. The exception is some congenital hernias and some hernias which occur due to pregnancy. An umbilical hernia will either stay the same, or with time may get larger. When the umbilical hernia becomes problematic, on occasion incarceration or strangulation may occur. In this case the patient will need emergency surgery to repair the hernia.

The resulting scar is the least noticeable of all hernia scars and frequently can be hidden in the umbilical region, as the "belly button" itself is a type of scar.

Rehab time and procedure is about the same as with inguinal hernias.

The Incisional Hernia

Incisional hernias occur in the abdominal wall where there was a prior surgical incision. Prior surgical incisions may be from a previous appendectomy, cholecystectomy, hysterectomy, or abdominal exploratory surgery. The hernias occur in this region as result of strenuous activities. It can also occur if the surgical incision was improperly closed, or if there was an infection present such as in the case of a ruptured appendicitis.

Another factor known to cause a weakening of the abdominal wall resulting in an incisional hernia is a decreased amount of collagen which affects the fascia or abdominal wall integrity. Diminished collagen and the resulting weakness in the abdominal wall have been known to be caused by poor diet, smoking, obesity, advancing age, and immune compromised patients. The main causes of immune compromise are cancer, AIDS, and chronic steroid use.

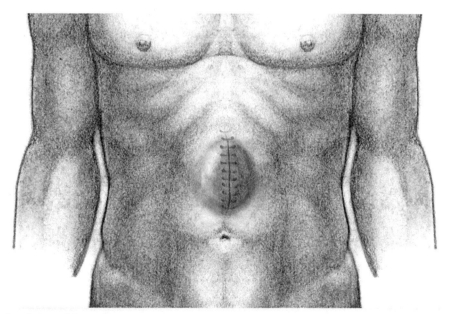

Incisional hernia

When an incisional hernia develops, similar to other hernias there is an accompanying swelling or bulge at the site of the incision. The contents of the hernia include the hernia sac or peritoneum as well as the intestines or omental fat.

Since a typical incisional hernia results from a prior incision that was repaired primarily without mesh, it is important that these hernias are repaired using a tension-free mesh technique. Tension-free mesh repairs will diminish the incidence of hernia recurrence.

Incisional hernias may be accompanied by pain. However, in most instances they are accompanied by the presence of a painless bulge.

Incisional hernias can be much larger in size than other hernias. While they usually begin as a one-inch hernia, they often increase in size— eventually becoming the same size as the incision. It is not unusual to see a 12-inch hernia in conjunction with a 12-inch incision scar.

When an incisional hernia occurs it is recommended that they are treated surgically soon after diagnosis because incisional hernias will almost always enlarge if not treated. The enlargement of an incisional hernia generally takes place over a period of a few months.

The resulting scar can be the same size as the original hernia, but it is usually about an inch or two larger than the hernia.

Although I encourage my patients to begin walking one day after incisional hernia surgery, the rehab is generally slower and takes longer than other hernias. This is due to the slow healing nature of scar tissue.

The Femoral Hernia

Femoral hernias present in the groin region and are similar to inguinal hernias. Femoral hernias occur in or below the crease between the thigh and the abdomen, whereas inguinal hernias occur above the thigh crease. This is a distinguishing factor between femoral and inguinal hernias. The femoral hernias protrude through a portion of the anatomy known as the femoral canal. Femoral hernias are much less common that inguinal hernias. Since femoral hernias are rare, they are frequently misdiagnosed as inguinal hernias.

It may be necessary to consult a hernia specialist to distinguish a femoral hernia from an inguinal hernia. If you suspect the presence of a femoral hernia, be sure to consult a physician because a femoral hernia almost always requires surgery on an urgent basis. Due to the narrowness in the femoral canal, the femoral hernia is more likely to become strangulated or incarcerated. Therefore, once the diagnosis of a femoral hernia is made

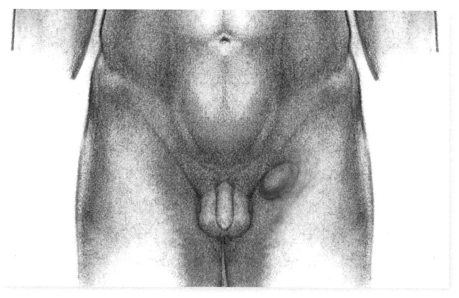

Femoral hernia

it is advisable to undergo surgical correction of the hernia without delay.

The scar after femoral hernia surgery is similar to that of an inguinal hernia, and the rehab is also similar to that of an inguinal hernia.

The Epigastric Hernia

Epigastric hernias occur in the midline of the abdominal wall between the xiphoid sternum or breast bone and the umbilicus or navel. Epigastric hernias are caused by a weakness in the upper abdominal wall. Epigastric hernias vary in size from a half inch to one inch. In rare instances they can become about three inches in size.

Although typically small in size, epigastric hernias tend to become painful because they contain a piece of fat which becomes pinched as it protrudes through the small hernia opening. When epigastric hernias begin to cause discomfort they should be surgically repaired. Over all, due to

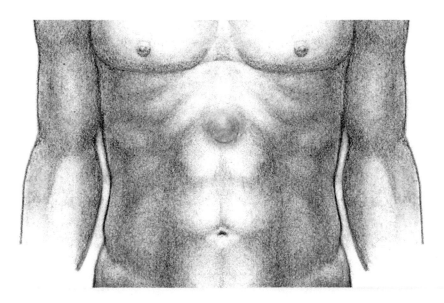

Epigastric hernia

their small size, these hernias are less likely to contain intestines or develop strangulation.

The resulting scar varies with the size of the hernia, but is generally one to three inches. Rehab is about the same as with an inguinal hernia.

The Ventral Hernia

A ventral hernia may occur anywhere in the abdominal wall. Umbilical hernias are a form of a ventral hernia as are epigastric hernias. The term "ventral hernia" refers to all abdominal wall hernias except for inguinal or femoral hernias. When the term "ventral hernia" is used to describe a hernia, it is not specific regarding the location of the hernia unless stated. For example, an upper abdominal ventral hernia is an epigastric hernia; and a mid abdominal ventral hernia is an umbilical hernia. A spigellian hernia is the name given to a ventral hernia that is located in the lower abdominal wall on either the

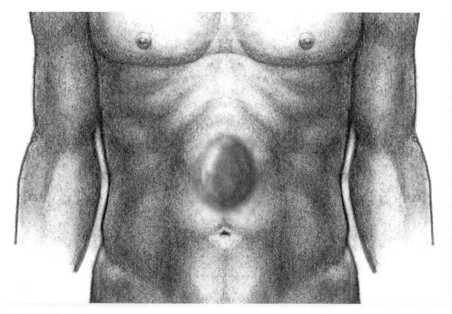

Ventral hernia

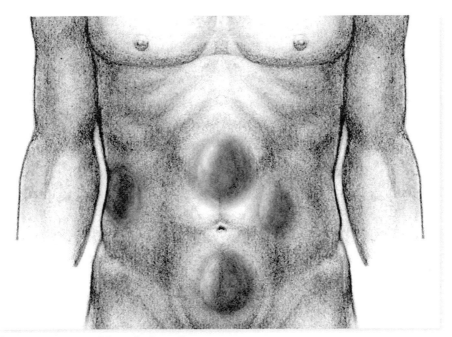

Common ventral hernia locations

right or left side.

Most commonly, ventral hernias occur in the midline but may also occur in the flank or sides. When an opening in the abdominal wall is present the fatty tissue or intestines will protrude. Ventral hernias occur as a result of a weakness or a tearing in the abdominal wall musculature due to increased pressure—typically from lifting or straining. Non strenuous activities, such medical factors as chronic constipation, urinary disturbances, or chronic cough, may also result in ventral hernias.

If a ventral hernia is untreated it may become as large as a grapefruit. Once diagnosed, a small ventral hernia does not require immediate surgery providing it does not cause pain. It can be merely observed by the patient over time. However once the hernia begins to enlarge, it should be immediately treated because a ventral hernia will almost always continue to enlarge. The larger a ventral hernia becomes, the operative repair becomes more difficult, complicated, and painful. Most ventral hernias contain large amounts of intestine and have a wide opening or neck. Because these hernias have a large neck or opening in the abdominal wall, they are less likely to become incarcerated.

The scar of a ventral hernia will usually be the same size or a little larger than the hernia itself. Rehab is very similar to an inguinal hernia.

The Incarcerated Hernia

All hernias are in danger of becoming incarcerated. The term refers to a hernia that cannot be reduced. Initially, most hernias are reducible—which means that they can be pushed back in. This usually is described by most patients as a "squishy" feeling. Some patients state that they have a bulge when standing, but at the end of the day it disappears when they lie in bed. This is a reducible hernia because the abdominal wall permits the contents of the hernia to return to the abdominal cavity.

With an incarcerated hernia, this no longer occurs—the contents of the hernia no longer will return into the abdominal cavity—because the abdominal contents within the bulge are too large to fit through the hernia opening in the abdominal wall.

Incarcerated hernias are very annoying. If you can, imagine how uncomfortable it would feel to have a balloon-shaped structure, or bag, attached to your outer body and containing your intestines.

I have seen far too many patients come to my office with large incarcerated hernias which initially started out as a reducible non-tender small hernia.

Incarcerated hernias have adequate blood flow to their contents, however surgery should be performed on an urgent basis before strangulation occurs.

The Strangulated Hernia

All hernias are in danger of becoming strangulated. This situation is similar to incarcerated hernias in that they are no longer reducible. When strangulation occurs, the blood flow to the contents of the hernia is impeded. At this point, the hernia and its contents are in danger of rupturing.

All strangulated hernias are very painful. Patients who develop a strangulated hernia are in danger of developing serious infections, gangrene—and in some extreme instances a strangulated hernia can lead to death of the patient.

When a strangulated hernia occurs, emergency surgery is of the utmost importance. Unfortunately strangulation can happen to any hernia without any warning.

CHAPTER FOUR

The Treatment of Hernias

Hernias require surgery. Without surgery hernias will not go away. A hernia will either stay the same or become larger over time. As the hernia enlarges it becomes more difficult for the hernia to be surgically repaired. The more difficult surgery results in the more protracted patient recovery. Repairing a small hernia is a much less complicated process than repairing a larger hernia. A larger hernia requires more time to perform the surgery, a greater number of sutures, a larger mesh, and consequentially a longer and often more painful recovery. Also, a greater number of postoperative complications can occur when the hernia becomes larger in size.

There are multiple surgical methods of repairing a hernia.

The Conventional Method.

The conventional method has been around since the turn of the 20th century. It utilizes the direct suture of the hernia defect without the use of a mesh. Using either the hands or special instruments, the surgeon pushes the protruding tissue, or the hernia, back into the abdominal cavity. Any hernia sac that is formed is either inverted in the abdominal cavity or removed by cutting it with a scalpel. The weakness or tear in the abdominal wall muscle is then repaired by sewing the surrounding muscle together with sutures.

Since there is tension in the wound after this method of surgery, the patient is placed on a weight lifting limit not to exceed 40 pounds after surgery. And since there is frequent tension in the wound as the patient goes about normal daily activities, this results in a prolonged healing time, on the average of 6 to 8 weeks. The conventional method results in more postoperative pain since the tissues are under constant tension. The recurrence rate is higher with the conventional method as compared to the methods of non tension using mesh.

The conventional method is used primarily in patients who have developed strangulated hernias, or who would face a high risk of infection if mesh were used.

The caveat of waiting too long for hernia surgery is that if the hernia becomes strangulated the end result is a less secure hernia repair since the strangulation requires emergency surgery without the use of mesh. Therefore the preferred treatment of a hernia is early surgery to avoid strangulation. I caution you to seek a second opinion if the surgeon you consult with recommends the conventional method when your hernia is not considered an emergency surgery situation.

The Tension-free Mesh Method.

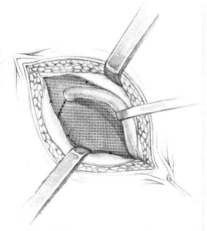
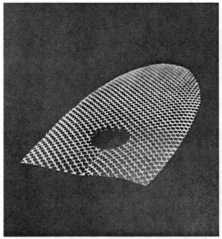

Hernia mesh technique for inguinal hernia surgery.

Hernia mesh

The tension-free mesh technique is the preferred method of hernia repair preformed by myself and most surgeons I know. This method has been in practice since the 1970s. At my Hernia Center the mesh is custom made to fit each patient. With the mesh technique not only is the defect in the abdominal wall repaired but the surrounding area of the groin is reinforced. This diminishes the chance of recurrent hernias.

There is a theory that hernias are the result of an inherent collagen based weakness of the abdominal wall. In other words, the abdominal wall of certain people who are prone to develop hernias is weaker compared to the population at large. Patients who have developed a hernia in the presence of this weakness are at risk of developing a recurrent hernia. By reinforcing the abdominal wall with mesh, the result is a strengthening of the abdominal wall and a reduced incidence overall of a hernia recurrence.

During this technique any protruding hernia sac is either excised or reduced into the abdominal cavity. Reduction of the hernia is done by simply pushing the hernia and its contents back into the abdominal cavity.

The tension-free mesh technique reduces the chance of recurrence to 0.5 percent or one in two hundred. However, in my practice the recurrence rate is 0.2 percent or one in five hundred. The tension-free method also provides patients with a shorter recovery time and greatly reduces postoperative pain. The tension-free technique involves the placement of a synthetic mesh in the inguinal region to repair and strengthen the abdominal wall. At my Hernia Center we use only the tension-free mesh technique and tailor the repair to the patient by selecting the appropriate mesh for each individual. With my technique there is no such thing as "one mesh fits all." Also, with this technique there is no unnatural tension. Consequentially, the patient will have less pain and a lower incidence of hernia recurrence. The mesh is customized after the incision is made and the hernia is exposed. The mesh is fashioned to cover the muscles of the inguinal region.

A flexible mesh is made of a non absorbable material. The mesh is sutured, glued or stapled in place. Over a period of a few weeks, it becomes incorporated by the surrounding tissues. The mesh effectively repairs the hernia and at the same time prevents recurrence. A lattice of fibrous tissue is deposited on the mesh which incorporates new tissue growth and results in a stronger hernia repair.

Since the mesh is thin it is very flexible. As it becomes incorporated by the body, over time it can no longer be felt. Because of its flexibility, It will not inhibit physical activity after surgery. By extending the edges of the mesh beyond the weakness or hernia tear, the mesh supports the surrounding tissue of the hernia. The mesh, when properly placed, will not separate from the muscle. This allows the patient to resume strenuous physical activity without fear of recurrence.

The tension-free mesh technique enables the surgeon to customize the repair. A large patient will obviously get a larger mesh than a patient who is smaller in size. A patient who requires a lot of flexibility, such as a runner, a tennis player, or a cyclist, will need a looser fitting mesh allowing additional movement. The looser mesh allows a speedier recovery due to more flexibility, thus allowing the patients to continue their activities with a minimum amount of pain. At the same time it minimizes the chance of hernia recurrence.

The type of patient who performs heavy strenuous work will require a reinforced mesh to allow maximum strength. This technique is used for a weightlifter, or a person whose work requires them to use a considerable amount of continuous muscle strain such as a laborer in shipping and receiving, or a construction worker. This type of reinforced hernia repair might initially be more painful requiring additional recovery time. But it also allows these patients to regain their ability to perform daily heavy work without fear of recurrence.

The Plug Technique.

The plug technique utilizes a variation of the tension-free mesh technique. In this technique a mesh plug is used to seal the opening of the hernia after it has been reduced. The plug seals or closes the hernia in a manner similar to corking a bottle. The plug repairs the hernia. An onlay mesh is then

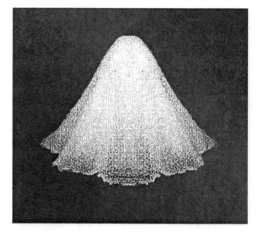

Hernia mesh plug and patch

used to blanket the abdominal wall in order to prevent a recurrent hernia. Not all surgeons suture the onlay mesh in place.

I do not perform this technique because the plug constricts and this can lead to nerve entrapment resulting in chronic groin pain, or spermaticord entrapment resulting in chronic testicular pain.

The Laparoscopic Method.

The laparoscopic method utilizes a video camera and a lighted tube which is inserted into a small incision in the abdominal wall. During the operation this lighted tube and camera allows the surgeon to find and repair the hernia. The laparoscopic method utilizes a mesh that is similar to the tension-free mesh technique. Therefore, the laparoscopic method is also a tension-free technique, with the difference being the mesh is placed on the *inner* side of the muscle defect—whereas with the tension-free method, the mesh is usually placed on the *outer* side of the muscle defect.

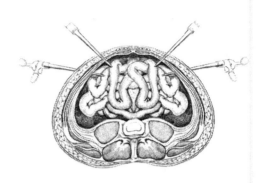

Laparoscopic surgery typically uses mesh which is stapled in place. The staples are placed using an instrument specially designed for this task. Usually the staples are made of stainless steel.

The laparoscopic method is not for everyone. It is not recommended to repair large or incarcerated hernias, or for patients with previous pelvic surgeries, or patients who cannot

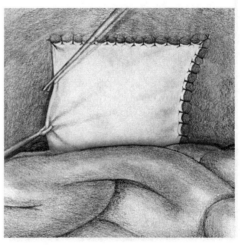

Laparoscopic method

tolerate general anesthesia. The laparoscopic technique is more costly than the tension-free mesh method, and may require slightly more time to complete the procedure.

With regards to recurrence or postoperative pain, overall there is no difference in the laparoscopic method and the open tension-free mesh technique. However, at the time of the writing of this book, I have seen multiple patients who have undergone the laparoscopic hernia repair then developed permanent chronic postoperative pain, and unfortunately have not been able to receive adequate treatment for their pain. At present there is no adequate method of treating these patients for their postoperative pain since the surgery is done internally. Whereas in using the open technique, if the patient develops postoperative pain, in most cases the surgeon is able to directly treat the patient's pain by either injection or by re-operating on the patient and freeing up or cutting the affected nerve. When the nerve is injured laproscopically, the nerve injury may not be apparent, plus the nerves are more difficult to treat due to their location.

Although the laparoscopic method is widely used, the only advantage I see is that the scar is slightly smaller. The laparoscopic method is more commonly used to treat multiple hernias and difficult recurrent hernias. I used to offer the option of laparoscopic surgery to my patients, but today I will only perform the open tension-free mesh technique. In my experience, the disadvantages of laparoscopic surgery far outweigh the advantages. The disadvantages of the laparoscopic hernia repair are:

1. General anesthesia is required.
2. The operation is more costly.
3. If a nerve injury occurs it is difficult to treat.
4. The scar formation resulting from laparoscopic hernia repair makes it more difficult to perform some vascular and prostate operations at a later date.

Chronic Pain After Hernia Surgery (Post Herniorrhaphy Pain Syndrome)

Patients who undergo hernia repair may develop a painful condition known as Post Herniorrhaphy Pain Syndrome. This condition affects 3 to 5 percent of all hernia patients. The cause of post herniorrhaphy pain syndrome can be determined by a thorough physical exam. An MRI neurography may be required to localize the injured nerve or neuroma, and to assist in determining the cause of the pain. An X-ray may be done to rule out a recurrent hernia or a missed hernia. X-ray is not always necessary prior to treatment of postoperative pain. Post Herniorrhaphy Pain Syndrome may be caused by a multiple of factors. These include: a missed hernia, a recurrent hernia, periostitis, constriction of the spermaticord, a neuroma, or an injured nerve.

A missed hernia is a hernia that was not repaired during surgery for any one of a number of reasons. For example, the patient may have been treated for a direct inguinal hernia but at the time of diagnosis the surgeon might have missed an indirect inguinal hernia. On the other hand, the surgeon may have repaired the indirect inguinal hernia and missed a direct inguinal hernia.

Unfortunately, I have seen it all. And sadly, this is often due to carelessness on the part of the physician.

An indirect inguinal hernia may be missed because it can be small and hidden in the spermaticord. It will not be seen unless the surgeon takes the time to explore this part of the anatomy of the inguinal canal. A surgeon repairing a large direct hernia may fail to do a complete intra-operative examination resulting in a missed hernia. Another common missed hernia is seen in patients with both femoral and inguinal hernias. If a patient has both an inguinal hernia and a femoral hernia, repairing only the inguinal hernia results in a persistent or missed femoral hernia.

A herniogram or an ultrasound is often helpful in assisting the surgeon with finding the missed or recurrent hernia. Also, a patient may develop a recurrent hernia after the original hernia repair surgery.

When the internal ring of the inguinal canal is repaired, constriction of the spermaticord may cause a painful testicle. If the blood supply to the testicle is diminished the testicle may become atrophic or decrease in size.

Periostitis occurs if deeply placed sutures breech the pubic bone or the fascia that is the covering of the pubic bone. When this occurs the sutures pull on the bone causing pain with movement.

Chronic pain after a surgery must be differentiated from unrelated or non hernia related causes of pain. For example, pain in a nearby structure or organ can be confused with post hernia pain. This includes the genital organs, the intestines, the pelvic bones, the pelvic organs, or the abdominal wall muscles.

The abdominal wall muscles can experience pain when the abdominal wall gets injured, resulting in a strained muscle. A muscle strain characteristically feels like nerve pain. However, a muscle strain will heal over time with or without treatment.

Chronic Pain due to Neuroma Formation

At the time of surgery the end of a cut nerve may develop a painful nerve ending known as a neuroma. Alternatively, rather than developing a neuroma the nerve may be damaged during a surgical procedure as a result of pinching or crushing. The damaged nerve also can cause pain in the same way as a neuroma causes pain.

The nerve may become painful if trapped by scar tissue. As the wound heals scarring occurs and at times the scarring entraps, pinches, or pulls the nerve resulting in postoperative pain. A nerve may also be trapped by misplaced mesh or a suture. As the wound heals mesh may contract, pulling on the nerve and leading to pain. A mesh plug may contract forming a meshoma. This contracting of the mesh plug may either entrap or exert pressure on a nerve causing pain.

Treatment of Chronic Pain Resulting from Hernia Surgery

Neuroma Surgery

The treatment of postoperative pain is dependent on the cause of the pain. When there is a recurrence or a missed hernia, then additional surgery is required to repair the hernia, as well as to alleviate the pain.

In treating a neuroma or a nerve injury, the first line of management is conservative. The patient should take oral pain medication. In addition, physical therapy may be required. If after a trial of oral medication pain persists, then local injection treatment may be instituted, consisting of a combination of a local anesthetic and corticosteroids. Generally the injections are instituted in a series of several injections in order to obtain pain relief. There are typically three separate sites where a nerve is injected. The two most common sites are at the location of the pain (also known as the trigger point) or along the effected nerve. In more resistant patients the nerve root may be injected close to the spine.

The results of conservative treatment are typically as follows: One third of the patients will receive partial relief of pain; one third will experience complete relief of pain; and one third of the patients will have no relief of pain whatsoever. Those patients who experience pain that is debilitating despite conservative therapy, which entails a combination of pain medication, physical therapy and injections, may require additional surgery. Surgery may be the only option available after a failed trial of conservation treatment and a waiting period of 6 to 12 months after surgery. At this time, if the patient still has a severe debilitating pain, then a repeat operation is performed to correct the ongoing cause of the pain.

Neuroma surgery, also known as neurectomy surgery, is utilized for chronic pain due to neuroma formation. The surgical treatment of postoperative nerve pain or neuroma is considered a serious undertaking and should be reserved for that patient who has persistent debilitating pain despite conservative measures. In some instances, prior to surgery, MRI neurography may be necessary to determine if a neuroma is present. In most cases the cause of the pain is determined by the surgeon during the operation.

There are three groin nerves which are known to cause pain after hernia surgery. It is possible to perform the surgery without first determining which nerve is the cause of pain. There are a variety of operations that can be preformed. Typically patients who have post hernia debilitating pain undergo a wound exploration. At the time of wound exploration the previous incision is explored and an attempt is made to determine the cause of the postoperative pain. The technique which I prefer is a wound exploration and a triple neurectomy in which all three groin nerves are divided and the nerve endings are ligated and buried in muscle tissue. Cutting the nerve interrupts the pain transmission by the nerve. Burying the nerve in the muscle tissue prevents the nerve from forming a neuroma.

There is an alternative method which I do not personally practice. This involves a wound exploration and instead of dividing all three nerves, the effected nerve (or nerves), which may be trapped are freed up. I do not find this to be a favorable method because a damaged nerve might continue to cause pain despite it being loosened or freed up. This is because the damaged nerve tissue may continue to send signals of chronic pain syndrome even after having been freed. Therefore I prefer the triple neurectomy in which the nerves are isolated and then divided. Even though the damaged nerve on inspection may have the same appearance as a healthy nerve, it can still cause pain. This is because the nerve, which is damaged, may heal within a painful scar.

Unfortunately the postoperative treatment of nerve pain is not always successful in alleviating the pain syndrome in every instance. Since the nerves are intentionally divided during this operation, some patients will experience an area of permanent numbness.

The typical recovery period after this surgery is between 4 to 6 weeks. The results of neurectomy surgery are as follows: 40% of patients will experience complete relief of pain; 40% of patients will receive partial relief of pain; 15% of the patients will have no relief of pain; and 5% of patients will not only receive no relief of pain, but the pain will actually become worse after the surgery.

Since I am a hernia specialist I am occasionally approached by general surgeons to correct their mistakes. It is unfortunate that when a mistake occurs the problem is often resolved with less than perfect results. When I perform hernia surgery I make it a point to protect the nerves from injury. My policy is, the best way to treat a nerve problem is to prevent it from happening in the first place. Thus, my goal is to prevent complications from occurring by performing hernia surgery correctly the first time.

CHAPTER FIVE

Diagnosis and Treatment of the Two Most Common Types of Hernias
Inguinal & Umbilical

In this chapter I will define the two most common types of hernias, the symptoms, the findings, and the type of treatments available.

Inguinal Hernia

Inguinal hernias are also known as groin hernias. An inguinal hernia occurs when there is a tear in the portion of the abdominal wall known as the inguinal canal. A bulge is created as the abdominal wall muscle tears. The abdominal wall contents which consist of either the intestines or fatty tissues protrude through the tear. This creates a bulge which is the hernia. Inguinal hernias are the most common type of hernias. Inguinal hernias or groin hernias are located between the lower abdomen and the upper thigh. They may occur on one side, or both the right and left side. When they occur on both sides they are called bilateral inguinal hernias.

In *males* inguinal hernias occur in the groin also known as the inguinal region because in this location the abdominal wall is weak as a result of the testes descending through the inguinal canal from the abdomen into the scrotum. By the passage of the vas deferens and the testicular arteries and veins, a natural weakness is created in the abdominal wall. This weakness

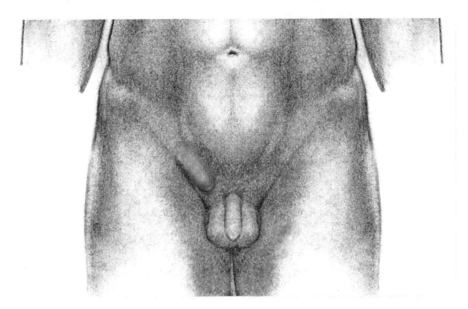

Inguinal hernia

results in more hernias developing in the inguinal location than any other locations. *Females* develop hernias in the same location due to the weakness created by the round ligament of the uterus with its accompanying vessels.

Symptoms of Inguinal Hernia

An inguinal hernia may present anywhere between very painful to completely painless. But most inguinal hernias tend to be relatively painless. More often, my patients simply complain of an unsightly bulge. Generally, the bulge is described as an "uncomfortable bulge that is not painful." Inguinal hernias appear while standing, walking, straining, or coughing; and will disappear while lying down. In time, hernias progressively increase in size and become more uncomfortable. Pain from a hernia may be referred (transmitted) to the leg, the back, or the genital regions.

When the hernia, which was previously non painful develops pain and an inability to reduce itself, the hernia may have become incarcerated.

Incarcerated hernias may develop into a medical emergency known as strangulation. When a hernia becomes either painful or difficult to reduce, it is important to seek medical attention as soon as possible.

Diagnosis of Inguinal Hernia

The diagnosis of an inguinal hernia can be made by a medical history and physical examination. It is not necessary to perform X-rays to diagnose this type of hernia. X-rays are usually reserved to diagnose rare types of hernias that are difficult to find. When the inguinal hernia is readily apparent, which is almost always the case, X-rays are not necessary.

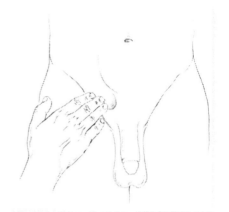

Examination of a an inguinal hernia patient

Causes of Inguinal Hernia

Inguinal hernias may be congenital or present at birth. Inguinal hernias can be acquired as a result of sudden or repetitive straining which results in an increase in abdominal pressure that weakens the abdominal wall. Straining occurs while performing such as lift pushing or pulling heavy loads at work. Athletes may develop hernias while training or in competition. Medical causes of hernias are the result of straining while passing urine, chronic coughing, or with constipation.

Treatment of Inguinal Hernias

Surgical treatment of inguinal hernias is necessary to repair them. Hernias will not go away or heal on their own. There is no medication, diet or exercise that will make a hernia go away. Any patient who claims to have had an inguinal hernia go away without surgery never had one in the first place. Most likely, what they really had was a muscle strain in the inguinal area. In my experience, the safest and most effective way to repair a hernia is with the tension-free mesh technique. This method is utilized for repairing inguinal hernias as well as many of the other types of hernias. Inguinal hernia surgery involves replacement of the contents of the hernia sac back to its normal location and closing the tear in the abdominal wall. There are several methods of accomplishing this. The tension-free technique involves placement of a synthetic mesh to both repair the hernia as well as to strengthen the abdominal wall. On the other hand, the conventional method relies on sewing the edges of the weak or torn muscles together without any type of reinforcement.

Conventional Method of Inguinal Hernia Repair

The conventional method of hernia repair which does not utilize mesh places undo tension on the wound. This method has a higher incidence of pain and a higher incidence of recurrence as compared to the open tension-free mesh technique. In addition, as compared to the conventional method, the tension-free mesh technique has not only less pain, but a shorter recovery period. Patients are able to return sooner to their jobs and other physical activities.

Open Tension-Free Method of Inguinal Hernia Repair

The open tension-free method is the only technique that I use to repair hernias. This technique uses a permanent mesh. The size of the mesh is tailor fitted for each patient depending on the size of the patient, their activities, and the location of the hernia. Some surgeons practice a "one size fits all" technique in which all hernias are fixed using the same size mesh. I have found that by performing a customized technique, tailor made for the individual, the hernia patient is able to resume their normal pre-injury activities with minimized recovery and pain.

Using the tension-free mesh technique, I avoid unnecessary tension in the wound, creating a more flexible wound. This allows for greater mobility during the recovery phase. The material that I use is a flexible Polypropylene mesh. This mesh is used to both repair the hernia and to reinforce the surrounding tissues preventing a recurrent hernia from developing. Once placed, the surrounding tissues of the abdominal wall form a lattice within the mesh adding strength to the abdominal wall and lessening the chance

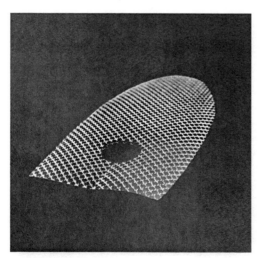

Hernia mesh

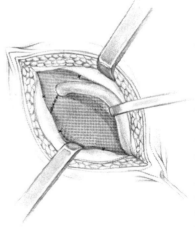

Hernia mesh technique for inguinal hernia surgery.

of recurrence. The mesh becomes incorporated safely and easily into the abdominal wall. The mesh is flexible and cannot be felt once fully incorporated.

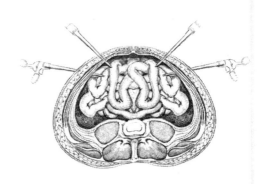

Laparoscopic Method of Inguinal Hernia Repair

The laparoscopic technique utilizes a flexible mesh and is also tension-free. This method uses a lighted tube and a video camera which enables the surgeon to perform the hernia repair.

I do not perform this operation because the benefits are minimal and disadvantages

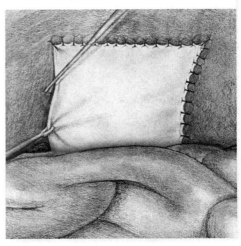

Laparoscopic method

are potentially serious. This operation is still in the developmental stages. I believe that once the operation has been fully developed there may be a benefit to this procedure. The primary advantage of laparoscopic hernia technique is in the repair of multiple hernias and in recurrent hernias.

Comparison of Open Tension-Free and Laparoscopic Method of Inguinal Hernia Repair

As of the writing of this book, the benefits of laparoscopic and the open tension-free mesh technique hernia repair are similar. The similarities of both operations include minimal postoperative pain, early return to work, and a small incision. Where they differ is regarding the complications. All hernia operations have potential complications.

1. The complications of laparoscopic surgery are bowel perforation which is unique to laparoscopic hernia surgery.

2. Complications related to general anesthesia which is required in laparoscopic hernia repair.

3. Chronic postoperative pain. Postoperative pain occurs with both open and laparoscopic hernia repairs. However postoperative pain is less resistant to treatment after laparoscopic surgery because the nerve damage is usually a result of internally placed staples which are inaccessible; and treatment protocols for corrective measures have not yet been written.

4. Recent medical journal articles report that surgeons are finding extreme difficulty in performing prostate surgery and vascular operations in the region which has been scarred by laparoscopic hernia repairs.

Methods of Anesthesia Used in Inguinal Hernia Repair

Inguinal hernia surgery may be performed under various types of anesthesia including local anesthesia by itself, local anesthesia with sedation, spinal anesthesia, or general anesthesia. I prefer to use local anesthesia with sedation. Utilizing this technique, patients are usually able to return home the same day and often require little to no pain medication. All patients are pre-screened for allergies

Local Anesthesia

The anesthesiologist starts an intravenous line. This is to ensure a safe operation. A local anesthetic is injected into the region of the surgery. The type of local anesthesia that is used consists of a combination of a long acting anesthetic such as Marcaine which is mixed with Lidocaine and Epinephrine. The Marcaine provides anesthesia for 4 to 6 hours. Lidocaine is a short acting local anesthetic. Epinephrine constricts the blood vessels and prevents bleeding during surgery. By using this combination, patients experience painless surgery, diminishing bleeding during surgery, and the recovery is quicker with low postoperative pain.

Local Anesthesia with Sedation

This is my preferred method of hernia repair for routine non complicated hernia patients. This entails the anesthesiologist starting an intravenous line. He or she then introduces a sedative and pain medication through the intravenous line.. A combination of medications is used during this technique. They include Versed, a sedative; Demerol, a narcotic for pain; and Propofol, a sedative. This combination used in hernia repair is similar to the medication given during a colonoscopy.

Once the patient has received the medication and is relaxed and pain free, local anesthetic is injected into the region of the surgery. This is similar to the local anesthesia mentioned in the above section entitled *local anesthesia*. The type of local anesthesia that is used consists of a combination of a long acting anesthetic such as Marcaine which is mixed with Lidocaine and Epinephrine. The Marcaine provides anesthesia for 4 to 6 hours. Lidocaine is a short acting local anesthetic. Epinephrine constricts the blood vessels and prevents bleeding during surgery. By using this combination, patients experience painless surgery, diminishing bleeding during surgery, and the recovery is quicker with low postoperative pain.

Although patients are only sedated, the majority of them will remain asleep throughout the operation. Patients usually awaken on their own as the anesthesiologist titrates the dosage of the medication to wear off by the end of the procedure. Sometimes the anesthesiologist awakens the patients in a manner similar to awakening a sleeping person without the use of additional medication.

Once they are awakened patients are taken to the recovery room. The patients will generally walk from the operating table to the recovery room because the short-acting sedative medication wears off quickly. Postoperatively, while the short acting local anesthetic medication has worn off, the long acting local anesthetic medication provides pain relief for several hours.

Sedation relaxes the patients. During the time the patients are on the operating table, they are either very relaxed or asleep. Due to the sedation they do not feel the pain effects of the needle at the time the local anesthetic is given. Following sedation, the surgery can be performed under local anesthesia. The local anesthesia method is preferred because patients are pain free, the procedure is safe, and there are a minimal amount of side effects.

General Anesthesia

The anesthesiologist starts an intravenous line. Patients are put to sleep using very strong medication. Unlike local anesthesia with sedation, a breathing tube is used to assist with respiration. We also use a local anesthetic which is injected into the region of the surgery.

Alternatively, with general anesthesia as compared to a local anesthesia, or local anesthesia with sedation, there are more potential side effects including sore throat, headaches, and nausea. Patients with a local anesthetic with sedation tend to have minimal disorientation and are able to recover quickly.

Post Operative Care

Patients are discharged the same day of surgery. They receive a prescription for pain pills. After a couple of days postoperatively, most patients may require either over-the-counter pain medication or no medication. A couple days after surgery they are able to return to their routine daily activities consisting of washing, dressing, going to the restroom, going to the kitchen for meals, walking, and finally driving. All patients will have temporary numbness in the region of the surgery. The numbness typically lasts four to six hours.

Umbilical Hernia

Umbilical hernias occur around the region known as the belly button, naval, or the umbilicus. The size of a hernia sac can vary between 1 to 4 inches in diameter. The hernia sac consists of peritoneum, and sometimes fatty tissue and intestines. The size of the neck of the hernia can also vary between 1 to 4 inches in diameter. The neck is a defect in the abdominal wall through

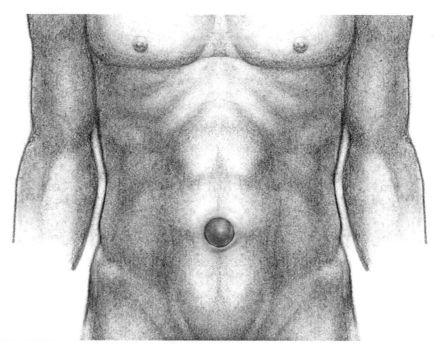

Umbilical hernia

which the hernia contents protrude. The larger a hernia the more likely it is to contain intestinal contents. The umbilical hernia occurs as a result of a tear in the abdominal wall lining through which abdominal organs or fatty tissue protrudes through.

Umbilical hernias can be acquired. In other words they may result from sudden or repetitive straining during which time the abdominal wall weakens and develops a hernia defect. However, umbilical hernias can also be congenital or present since birth. The congenital umbilical hernias occur at birth when the umbilical ring from which the umbilical cord exits does not quite heal, therefore leaving a defect in the naval. Infants that are born prematurely are more likely to develop an abdominal wall hernia than a full term infant. Small infant hernias may close on their own by age five. However, when the infant reaches age five, if the hernia is still present it will not close on its own. Large congenital umbilical hernias will not close without surgery.

Likewise, adult umbilical hernias will not heal without surgery. One exception is female patients who develop hernias as a result of pregnancy may heal without surgery.

When an umbilical hernia is not surgically repaired it will eventually get larger as the surrounding abdominal muscles become weaker. This creates an appearance of the navel like an "outie" instead of an "innie." A patient will notice a protruding bulge in her or his umbilical region. Although it is possible, umbilical hernias rarely strangulate or incarcerate.

The signs and symptoms of an umbilical hernia vary from person to person. The primary symptom is that of a soft, squishy bulge in the navel region. This bulge may be pushed in but shortly after protrudes outward on its own. Umbilical hernias might be accompanied by pain, but pain is not always present. The pain associated with an umbilical hernia is usually present during straining activities such as lifting, coughing, or sneezing. If the hernia becomes red or swollen, there is the possibility of an incarcerated or strangulated hernia, which requires emergency surgery. Without surgery the umbilical hernia will not go away. The hernia may stay the same, enlarge, or become incarcerated. I recommend that these hernias be repaired at the soonest possible convenience even in the non emergency patients.

Treatment of Umbilical Hernias

There are many techniques available for repairing umbilical hernias. Hernia repair consists of a closure of the abdominal wall defect.

The conventional method entails closing the abdominal wall with sutures and overlapping muscle. This non mesh technique may create a considerable amount of tension in the wound. This method is used on very small hernias, usually less than 2 cm.

The most commonly practiced method of repairing an umbilical hernia is the mesh or plug technique. This method entails placing a plug or the tension-free mesh. Using the tension-free mesh technique, the weakness of

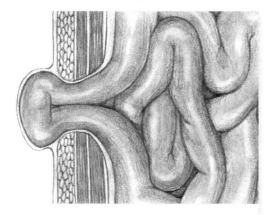

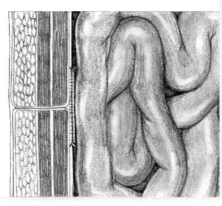

the abdominal wall through which the hernia is present is remedied.

Surgery is performed by making an incision in the area of the hernia, replacing the protruding abdominal contents back into the abdominal cavity and repairing the hernia. At the same time, the surrounding abdominal muscles are reinforced using a permanent flexible non absorbable mesh. The mesh is typically placed behind the muscles and in front of the peritoneal cavity

Treatment of umbilical hernia using mesh technique.

being separated from the peritoneal cavity by a layer called the peritoneum. In certain instances, when the peritoneal cavity has been violated, there is available a non adhesive mesh which when in contact with the abdominal contents is less likely to form postoperative adhesions.

The safest and most effective way to repair an umbilical hernia is the tension-free mesh technique. The procedure is performed as a one day outpatient procedure, typically under local anesthesia with sedation. The hernia mesh is placed behind the hole in the abdominal wall. The size of the mesh is tailored depending on the size of the individual and the size of the hernia. This mesh is incorporated by the body tissues as new growth forms around the mesh and creates a supportive lattice strengthening the abdominal wall muscles. Using this technique the muscles are not cut, nor are they sutured together. This flexible thin polypropylene mesh incorporates itself safely with the muscles of the abdominal wall.

Most patients feel little to no discomfort as they return to daily activities. The end result is minimal or no restrictive postoperative movements. Almost all patients are highly satisfied with this technique that provides them with a fast return to everyday life with no or minimal postoperative pain. With a properly performed tension-free technique, there is a minimization of postoperative pain problems with an extremely low recurrence rate. You'll be returning to your regular activities sooner with fewer or no postoperative restrictions.

Female Cosmetic Concerns

The following is a conversation between me and a female patient with an umbilical hernia. She was concerned about both hernia recurrence and the cosmetic appearance of the scar following surgery:

Patient: *Will I develop another hernia?*

Doctor Albin: It can happen, but it is extremely rare. When I repair the hernia, I use the tension-free mesh technique to not only repair the hernia but to reinforce the surrounding areas and diminish the chance of recurrence.

Patient: *What may occur if I wait to have my surgery later?*

Doctor Albin: If you wait to have your surgery later, your hernia may become incarcerated and you will need emergency surgery. A critical factor in an emergency is that the hernia is rapidly repaired. There is less emphasis on preventive surgery. Therefore, in an emergency situation, you have a higher chance of getting a hernia recurrence than you would expect in an elective surgery.

Patient: *I know it's not that bad now, however, when it's distended, it doesn't look that great. But what am I looking at as far as scarring. I like having a bare midriff and I'm concerned—might the scar look worse than the hernia?*

Doctor Albin: I would repair the hernia using a semi-circular incision within the belly button. The scar would have the appearance of a normal belly button wrinkle and would be easy to mask with cosmetics, if you feel it is necessary. But most likely, no one will ever notice you had surgery. The surgery takes a little longer. I am very experienced in a technique called key-hole surgery whereby the hernia is effectively repaired through a very small scar.

Note: I performed her operation through a key-hole incision. The scar was barely noticeable. It was one inch in length. The scar could only be seen at about 12 inches away from the patient. The patient was happy with her results. She said that she would be wearing a bikini to the beach this summer.

The issue of a noticeable scar is of particular concern to women in the film/TV and modeling industries. However, I have even had some male patients, especially professional bodybuilders, who are concerned about a scar that might show in a camera close-up. Fortunately there is "concealer" makeup (such as MAC Studio Finish), that comes in various skin shades, and is very effective in disappearing a scar, even at close range.

CHAPTER SIX

Pre-Op & Post Op Instructions / Recovery

PRE-OP:

Preparation for Surgery

The day before surgery do not take any food or drink by mouth after midnight. It is important to have an empty stomach at the time of surgery. Do not take aspirin one week prior to surgery as this may cause bleeding after surgery. Do not smoke, drink alcohol or chew gum as this may stimulate the body to produce intestinal juices, and may act as though the stomach is full. This could cause vomiting during surgery.

If you are told by your physician to take medication prior to surgery, such as medication for blood pressure, you may do so with a small sip of water. Children under the age of 18 must be accompanied by a parent or a legal guardian. You need to arrange transportation for your return home as you will not be able to drive yourself after surgery.

- The day of surgery you should arrive to the surgery center at least one hour prior to your appointed surgery time.
- The day of surgery take a shower and wash your hair, since you will find it uncomfortable to shower during the first couple postoperative days.
- Remove all nail polish from your fingernails. This is necessary because fingernails are used to monitor the oxygen level to your body during surgery.

- Do not use any adhesives on your dentures since they may be removed prior to the operation.
- Do not shave the surgical site as this will be done by the staff prepping you for the surgery.
- Wear loose fitting comfortable clothing which will be easily be taken off and put back on after surgery.
- Bring all the medication with you that you are currently taking so the surgeon as well as the anesthesia staff will be able to review them.
- Do not wear jewelry, or bring any valuables, large amounts of cash, or suitcases.

A pre-operative work up is necessary for all patients undergoing surgery. All patients are required to have a pre-operative history and physical examination. This is usually done at the time of your initial consultation. Be sure to bring with you, or have the names of, all the medications that you are taking.

Pre-operative laboratory testing is not necessary for all patients. A young healthy adult does not require any laboratory tests.

Your doctor will determine if any additional testing is necessary.

If you have a major medical problem you may be referred to a medical internist or a cardiologist prior to surgery.

Typically patients over the age of 40 will have an electrocardiogram.

In some instances the doctor may order a blood test. The blood test commonly requested includes a CBC, blood chemistry, a coagulation profile, and a urine analysis. These tests screen for a large number of medical problems, some of which include testing for infection, anemia, diabetes, kidney or urine problems.

In the case of fertile females, it is important to perform a pregnancy test.

POST-OP:

Travel After Surgery

At my surgery center I perform surgery on patients who have traveled from all over the United States, as well as the world. Since hernia surgery is minimally invasive, patients may travel by car one or two hours after surgery.

I do not advise flying until one day after surgery. Those patients who are going to take an airplane flight should have a postoperative checkup with their physician prior to departing.

Patients who are traveling by car the same day of surgery should limit their ride to 1 to 4 hours. Patients cannot drive themselves the day of surgery because the drugs they will be given during the surgery by the anesthesiologist will impair their driving. It is actually illegal to drive home the day of your surgery due to the drugs that will be in your system. Those patients who require further travel distance are advised to stay an additional day and have a post-op visit one day after surgery with their physician.

If the patient cannot find a friend or relative to drive them, they can take a taxi home. I provide my patients with pain medication so that they do not have to make stops on the way home. I recommend that my patients stock up on easily digestible food prior to surgery. Although many patients feel well and pain free after surgery, it is not a good idea to stop at a restaurant after surgery. This temporary good feeling is the result of the anesthetic drugs in the system. When they wear off the results can sometimes be a rather severe pain. I therefore advise going directly home after surgery.

What to Expect the First Few Days After Surgery

It is advisable, although not required, that the hernia patient has someone to spend the night with them after surgery. It is also advisable for the first 24 hours after surgery that patients stay in bed, and apply an ice pack to the surgical site (5 to 10 minutes every 30 minutes to one hour, while awake). It is permissible for the patient to walk to the dining table or the bathroom, but not much farther than that the day of surgery. I recommend that patients consume at minimum of two quarts of liquid following surgery. This helps to eliminate the anesthetic medication. Also I advise that they eat soup or a bland diet the rest of the day after surgery in order to avoid anesthetic related vomiting.

Your recovery period depends on multiple factors including the location of the hernia, the type of hernia, the repairing technique, as well as each individual's overall health. With the tension-free mesh technique the recovery period is considerably less than the conventional method without mesh. I typically see patients return to everyday activities within just a few days after surgery.

Everyday activities include dressing, bathing, walking, general self-hygiene and even driving a car. Most patients are able to return to this "normal" state within 2 to 3 days after surgery. In general, patients can return to light work, light recreational activity, and light sports activity in one to two weeks. However, they will not in every instance be at their pre-injury level. The more complex hernias such as bilateral, recurrent, or incisional hernias usually require a longer recovery period. The amount of recovery time with regards to these patients as a general rule is approximately 50% more than the simple routine hernias as previously described.

Food

It is important to maintain a healthy diet after surgery. Following surgery, be sure to drink an abundant amount of liquids in order to maintain hydration.

I recommend that you drink 8 glasses or two quarts of water, juice, or Gatorade. Due to the use of strong anesthetic drugs it is important to eat light the day before surgery; and to eat *nothing* after midnight the day of surgery.

After surgery you may start by eating small portions of easy digestible foods such as soup, rice, or over-boiled vegetables, or ground meat. This will diminish the incident of postoperative nausea and vomiting which anesthetic medications can cause. One day after surgery you may eat anything that agrees with your stomach.

Activities

The rest of the day following your surgery, it is recommended that the hernia patient remain in bed. It is permissible to walk to the bathroom or to the table for meals. It is important that the patient remain in bed and ice the wound for 5 to 10 minutes every 30 minutes to an hour while awake. Ice should be applied to the surgical wound for the first 24 to 48 hours to diminish postoperative swelling and pain. Do not put ice directly on the skin. Always put a layer of cloth between the ice and your skin. You can make several ice packs by filling plastic sandwich bags with water and placing the bags in the freezer. A bag of frozen peas also makes a good ice pack. The reason I recommend icing the wound is to prevent postoperative swelling.

Patients should strive to walk at least one hour a day starting the first day after surgery. By the second day after surgery this can be increased to two hours in divided amounts.

A simple guide to follow would be to walk within the house the first day after surgery. The second day after surgery, patients can walk outside of the house. For those patients who are feeling well enough by the third day after surgery, it's okay to leave their home and go for a short drive. Patients may drive themselves as long as they are not taking any medications that might impair them.

While walking it is important to maintain an erect, upright posture. Some patients tend to stoop because of the pain. The stooping posture can be corrected by looking in a full length mirror to ensure that you have the right walking posture. Improper walking or stooping may result in temporary back pain.

After the first day of surgery it is important *not* to remain in bed. Patients should either walk, or sit in a comfortable chair. If you feel the need to relax in bed, or take a nap, it is permissible. But take only one nap during the day. Lying in bed the entire day will increase the chance of getting blood clots in the legs. When a person is not moving their legs, blood can stagnate and form a blood clot. Non surgical common causes of leg blood clots are sitting for prolonged hours in an airplane, or lying in a hospital bed for days. In order to prevent this from occurring, I recommend ambulating my patients. Patients who are not ambulatory are advised to contract their calf muscles to prevent stagnation of blood in the leg veins. Overweight patients tend to be more prone to the development of this problem because they are less likely to ambulate.

Constipation

It is not uncommon for patients to develop constipation after surgery. Constipation is a result of pain that will be accentuated by straining. In addition, many of the pain medications are known to cause constipation. For this reason I recommend a high fiber diet and a stool softener after surgery. Those patients who require more than one prescription of pain medication should take stool softeners. If patients are unable to move their bowels by the second postoperative day, I recommend prune juice or a gentle laxative. By the third day, if constipation is still present then you should call your physician to prescribe a stronger laxative.

Wound Care

Keep your dressing dry and intact. It is normal to experience pain and slight swelling and redness at the wound site. Occasionally there might be a small draining or discharge of blood during the first 1 or 2 days postoperatively. If the swelling and the redness continue beyond a few days, and you develop an increasing discharge, you should consult your physician.

After surgery you should resume all your regular medications in addition to the medication that has been prescribed to you by your hernia surgeon. With most patients I recommend showering with removal of the dressing in five days. In some instances such as large hernias or complex hernias the dressing may need to remain in place for a week, depending on the type of hernia surgery. You should consult your physician in regards to dressing changes. I recommend cleaning the surgical wound initially with tap water. After five days, I advise tap water with a gentle diluted soap. I do not recommend scrubbing the wound with soap or applying iodine, alcohol or mercurochrome.

When To Call Your Surgeon After Surgery

You should call your physician if you develop any of the following symptoms:

- Difficulty urinating.
- Severe constipation (call if you are constipated for three days).
- Fever of 101 degrees Fahrenheit or greater.
- The incision becomes infected as evidenced by redness, increasing pain, swelling, or the development of a foul smell or a discharge.
- The incision opens or bleeds.
- If you feel overly sleepy, dizzy, or groggy.
- If you develop an allergic reaction to the pain medication. Allergic reactions include nausea, vomiting, redness, or a rash.

Some patients cannot tolerate stronger pain medications because of stomach sensitivity and may have to change the pain medication to an over-the-counter one that is less irritating, for example, Motrin, Advil, or Tylenol. Certain individuals who are hyper sensitive to pain may require additional care.

If the patient is having trouble sleeping due to pain the first 2-3 days, I recommend that they consult their physician. In this case, there may be some misunderstanding of the postoperative instructions.

Return to Work

Most patients have the ability to self-diagnose their ability to return to work. If they are experiencing minimal discomfort they can resume work. But they should make a point to avoid painful situations. Working in the face of severe pain may result in a setback and a delayed recovery. If you listen to your body it will tell you what you are allowed to do. One of the possible complications of returning to work in the first few days after surgery can be postoperative bleeding. Therefore it is advised that you be careful and avoid any potentially painful situations. Hernia recurrence in the initial postoperative period is very rare unless the patient performs very heavy lifting shortly after surgery.

With the tension-free mesh technique, the return to work can be expedited as a result of minimal postoperative pain. In order to access the ability of a patient to return to work, I have written a guide for the general population of routine hernia patients. However, please be aware that the ability to return to work will vary based on the respective physiology and the activity level of each patient. Furthermore, always consult with your physician for the time-table he or she recommends in your particular case.

RECOVERY:

Dr. Albin's Return to Work Guide:

Sedentary work: Sedentary work includes secretarial work, computer work, phone or office work. Sedentary work involves sitting, standing, and/or walking with lifting of less than 20 pounds. Patients can return to work 3 to 5 days after surgery. They will however continue to experience minimal pain which can be treated with over-the-counter pain medications such as Advil, Tylenol, or Motrin. These are the recommended pain medications because they will not impair the patient's ability to concentrate, work light machinery, or drive a car. These medications will serve to take the painful edge off the surgery.

Minimal to moderate physical work: This work includes electricians, plumbers, factory workers, mechanics, retail workers, and laborers, who occasionally lift up to or between 20 and 40 pounds. This does not include workers who repeatedly lift throughout the course of their work day. Usually these workers can return to unrestricted work within 2 weeks of surgery. They can actually return to work within one week with the light duty restriction of "no lifting over 20 pounds." On returning to work the patient will experience minimal pain that can be treated with over-the-counter pain medication such as Tylenol, Advil, or Motrin.

Heavy physical strenuous work: This work includes warehouse stockers, construction workers, road workers, and heavy duty mechanics. Patients can return to unrestricted work usually within 4 weeks after their surgery. They can also return to work within 1 week with a light duty restriction of "no lifting over 20 pounds." Or, these patients can return to work within 2 weeks with the restriction of "no lifting over 40 pounds; or no repetitive lifting." On returning to work they will experience minimal pain which can be handled with over-the-counter medication such as Tylenol, Motrin, or Advil. Additionally, to alleviate the pain, it is helpful to take warm soaks or warm baths shortly after returning home from work.

Very heavy physical strenuous work: The patients who have very strenuous work where they are continuously lifting, pushing and pulling heavy loads throughout the course of the day will return to regular work within 4 to 6 weeks.

The criteria for returning to work or other activities are based upon the pain associated with surgery, and not due to the integrity of actual hernia repair. The use of the tension-free mesh technique strengthens the abdominal wall approximately four times of that of a normal abdominal wall. The actual surgery, although not completely healed, maintains the integrity of the abdominal wall in the immediate postoperative period. Although theoretically a post hernia patient can typically perform heavy strenuous activities without rupturing the repair, I do not recommend this. In addition to being painful, there is the danger of causing bleeding in the surgical site. For this reason, during the first postoperative week of the healing process, I recommend that patients minimize their strenuous activities and instead go for long, daily walks. Walking assists in increasing the flexibility of the patient and diminishes the postoperative pain.

Returning to Recreational or Athletic Activity

I recommend to my patients that they return to recreational and athletic activity soon after surgery. Their ability and readiness to return to recreational activity depends on the type of hernia and the type of operation performed. As each patient is a unique individual, it is advisable to have a physician tailor your progressive return to recreational and athletic activities to fit your individual needs and abilities. I prefer to follow a four week regimen with regards to most athletes in the postoperative period.

- *Week #1*: primarily lighter easy activity such as walking and minimal stretching.
- *Week #2*: minimal to moderate activities. A long easy warm-up followed by an easy activity lasting 20 to 30 minutes.
- *Week #3*: moderate activity. A long easy warm-up followed by a moderate activity lasting up to an hour. This activity should be midway in intensity between a minimal and strenuous activity.
- *Week #4*: strenuous and physical activities. The usual warm-up followed by 75 to 85 percent of your typical physical activity.
- *Week #5 to #6:* Patients should be able to exercise at nearly their pre-injury state. I recommend that patients perform the activities 3 to 4 times a week with resting for one day in-between each active day.

Again, it is important to have a physician tailor the best program with regards to your returning to recreational and athletic activity. I highly recommend that the patient consult the operating surgeon to determine what will be the most effective program for you. To follow are general guidelines for the most common sports.

Runners: *One day* after surgery I advise my patients to walk one hour per day.

After *two or three* days I increase their walking up to two hours a day.

After my patients are very comfortable walking, then I will initiate running.

Typically I have the patient begin running *one week* postoperatively. Running activities

are performed in 5 minute intervals. Patients can run for 20 to 40 minutes divided by four to eight 5 minute intervals. The amount of minutes they run depends on their comfort level. This a typical running schedule for my patients:

The first full week of running usually begins in the *second postoperative week*. I recommend that patients initially run at the pace of a light jog.

- *Day one* includes five minute intervals during which time the patient will jog for one minute, followed by four minutes of walking.
- *Day two* is a day off running.
- *Day three* includes light jogging for an interval of two minutes, followed by three minutes of walking. This completes a five minute set, and the patient is advised to do four to eight similar sets.
- *Day four* is a day off running.
- *Day five* consists of an interval of three minutes of jogging, followed by two minutes of walking.
- *Day six* is a day off running.
- *Day seven* consists of light jogging for an interval of four minutes, followed by one minute of walking.

This completes the *first week* of running exercise. A similar interval schedule is used for the remaining weeks, however the pace can be stepped up from light jogging to moderate jogging.

On *week three* the pace can be increased from moderate jogging to a slow run.

By the *fourth week* I recommend that patients can run at their normal running pace.

By the *fifth week* there are no restrictions and they can do speed work, or run on hills as tolerated. If during this period the patient feels pain, I recommend that they take a couple days off.

During the *first month* of running I recommend that my patients continue with one minute rest during the five minute interval of time. This gives the body time to recover itself.

This program is to be used only as a guideline. I always advise my patients to avoid over exertion. For instance, it is acceptable to feel a certain amount of discomfort. When the patient is experiencing pain I recommend that they stop this activity. If they are to continue the activity in the presence of excessive pain for a prolonged period of time, their recovery period will be prolonged and this may cause a lighting up of their injury. This will not be considered a surgical complication, but it will result in a delayed recovery.

For example, let's say a distance runner who has run for 3 or 4 miles and is 1 or 2 miles from their destination experiences severe pain. I recommend that at this stage of the exercise they stop running and walk to the final destination. The severe pain will usually resolve and they can continue with their program.

Patients are told that this program is only a guideline and their ability to complete the program will differ depending on their individual abilities and overall health. Patients who are exceptionally healthy can complete the 4 week program within a 3 or a 3 ½ week period. Those who find they require more time may take 5 or 6 weeks. It is, however, rewarding to know that even if the patient doesn't complete the program within four weeks, they may be 75% to 85% recovered at that time.

Cyclists: *One day* after surgery I recommend that cyclists walk for an hour a day, and after 2 or 3 days increase their walking distance to 2 hours per day.

By *day three* they may begin cycling on a stationary bike. The stationary cycling should be done at a slow and low intensity, and should continue as such for the *first week*.

The *first week* cycling should be no more than 30 minutes a day. Gradually the cycling time may be increased up to a one hour period. I prefer that you use a stationary bike during the *first week* of recovery to avoid potential falls and injuries to the surgical site.

By *week two*, cyclists may ride on a non stationary bike. Initially I recommend that you bike on a flat terrain.

The first outdoor bike ride should be short. In the beginning, try riding for only twenty minutes outdoors. Add twenty minutes to your ride every other day. Gradually as your comfort level improves you may add additional time on the bike.

By *week three* it is acceptable to add some hills and speed work.

By *week four* you may cycle without restriction.

Since mountain bikers tend to take occasional hard falls, I recommend that they follow the "Cyclist" routine with the following distinctions: Initially they should bike on well cleared trails such as fire roads. It is advisable that they avoid situations where they might take a fall for the *first four weeks* after surgery. By the *fifth week* after surgery they should be well enough to ride at their pre-injury level.

Weightlifters: Starting *one day* after surgery I recommend walking for one hour per day.

After *two to three days* this is increased to 2 hours per day.

By *day five*, a patient may make his first trip to the gym. Patients may use light free weights or machines at minimal tension. This is done primarily to maintain the flexibility of the exercise without lifting weight. The maximum lifting during this period should not exceed 40 pounds for the *first month* postoperative. Use your toning weight as a guide.

Postoperative *week four* you may lift 25% of your toning weight.

Week five you may lift 50% of your toning weight.

Week six you may lift 75% of your toning weight.

Week seven you may lift 100% of your toning weight.

Week eight postoperatively you may begin lifting without restriction.

Pain should be used as a guideline. I recommend that patients who develop pain while lifting take one or two days off and resume their lifting activities at a lesser level or with a lesser amount of weight. I also recommend that the weightlifting is done at a maximum of *three to four times a week*.

Additionally, patients who lift without using trunk or core muscles may resume weightlifting during the *second postoperative week*. Trunk or core muscles are those muscle groups *not* involving the upper extremity or the lower extremity. While lifting using the extremities, I advise that during the *earlier period*, patients use machines rather than free weights.

Those patients who return to early weightlifting are able to do so without endangering their surgical repair. However, I advise that they are vigilant during this period and lift with moderation. The early lifting should not exceed the toning weight. My goal during this period is that my patients will maintain their strength and flexibility. This is not a strength gaining period, but a period in which they can recover from surgery and still maintain their overall strength without losing their extremity strength.

Golf: *One day* after surgery I recommend walking one hour per day.

After *two to three days* the walking is increased to 2 hours per day.

Day three patients may begin putting and chipping.

By *day five* you may be ready for a "pitch and put" round of golf, or par 3 golf courses. During this early postoperative period restrict yourself to irons greater than number 7. If you would like to work on the driving range it is better to concentrate on the short portion of the game.

By the end of the *second week* you may utilize the lower number irons.

Week three you may add the woods, and may also be ready for a 9-hole or executive golf course.

Week four you may play a full round of 18 hole golf without restriction. At this period you may not be at your pre-operative level. You might be 75% to 85% of your natural playing ability. If during this period there is difficulty with your swing I would advise a warm bath and stretching to increase flexibility. The best time to stretch is typically after the body has warmed up, such as at the end of a warm shower or at the end of an exercise.

Hiking: *One day* after surgery I recommend walking one hour per day on city sidewalks.

After *two to three days* the walking is increased to 2 hours per day.

Week one you may begin hiking on a flat terrain. I recommend that you start with a short easy hike. Gradually you may increase the distance and elevation depending on your comfort level. Hike sensibly and let someone know where you are going. Bring an ample amount of water and stay on the trail. Avoid hiking in terrain where you will be in danger of falling down.

On the *second week* you may begin with short, moderate hikes or long easy hiking.

Week three you may begin long moderate hikes.

Week four you may begin strenuous hikes.

Basketball: *One day* after surgery I recommend walking one hour per day.

After *two to three days* the walking is increased to 2 hours per day.

Day three postoperatively you may start shooting hoops by yourself. But keep it simple and mostly close range shots.

After *one week* try a one-on-one game with an opponent who will give you an easy game.

Week two you may play a full court game, but be prepared to sit out most of the game.

Week three you should be able to play a good portion of the game.

By *week four* you should be able to play a full court basketball game without restriction.

Tennis: *One day* after surgery I recommend walking one hour per day.

After *two to three* days the walking is increased to 2 hours per day.

By *day five* you may start hitting some tennis balls. Rally with an opponent who will hit the ball directly to you. It is not advisable at this early stage that you run after the balls. If the opponent cannot hit the ball directly to you, then your opponent is going to have to spend more time chasing after your missed balls. Thus, during this period you are essentially hitting balls that are coming right toward you, and working on your swing. I would also recommend during this period that you spend more time volleying with the ball, and that you do not practice overhead slams, or serve the ball with full force. Alternatively you can use a ball machine.

Week three you should play a game with minimal running.

By *week four* you should be able to play a game without restriction.

Summary of Returning to Recreational or Athletic Activity

On average, at *four weeks* after surgery, most athletes may return to recreational or athletic activities at full or near-full capacity, with the exception of weightlifting and contact sports. These sports require an additional recovery period.

Keep in mind that although you are returning within four weeks to your recreational activities, you *may not* be at a 100% level. Rather you might be at 75% to 85% of your skill level. It is normal to experience discomfort when returning to these recreational activities. However, if you are experiencing pain in this recovery process it is advisable that you stop those activities for awhile. Take a few days off, and when you return to the recreational activities, try a lower level of intensity. If you still have pain I recommend that you consult your physician.

CHAPTER SEVEN

Post Surgical Pain

One of the most frequent questions I get asked is, "After hernia surgery will I have pain?"

The short answer. All surgery is painful. The prescription pain medication is there to minimize the pain. You will most likely need to take it for the first few days. It takes 2 to 3 days of recovery before you can return to your normal daily activities. For a few days after surgery you will have a discomfort lasting one to two weeks, which is usually alleviated by over-the-counter pain medication. It is not unusual to experience an occasional twinge of pain up to one year after surgery.

The long answer. The average patient that I operate on will take 6 to 8 prescription pain pills postoperatively. I prescribe either Vicodin, Tylenol with Codeine, or Darvocett. Before they are released, I give my patients pain pills so that they do not have to stop at a pharmacy on the way home.

Beginning of week one after surgery:

The majority of my patients take prescription pain pills over the first 2 to 3 days only. Fifteen percent of my patients take zero or less than six pain pills.

Ten percent of my patients go through multiple pain prescriptions because of poor pain tolerance. Rather than using the prescribed pain pills, I encourage my patients to use over-the-counter medication such as Advil, Motrin, or Tylenol. The pain period with the most severity is 2 to 3 days postoperatively.

Patients can usually return to normal activities in two to three days after surgery. Return to normal activities entails dressing oneself, going to the bathroom, and sitting at the dinner table without assistance. Also, being able to exit the house, going for short walks, and driving a car. Patients who experience more pain return to normal activities in about 4 days, but rarely longer than 5 days. If you are unable to have this type of freedom of movement within 5 days you should consult your physician. In some cases, we find that those patients are not cooperating with the physician's instructions and are developing early wound stiffness. When this occurs I recommend taking multiple warm 15 minute baths a day, and begin stretching exercises to increase the flexibility and allow pain-free mobility.

Two to three days after surgery, most patients are able to go about their routine activities without the need of their prescription pain medication. Although they still experience mild to moderate pain during this period of time, the intensity of pain is not strong enough in severity that they require any medication except for Tylenol or a similar over-the-counter pain medication. Even though the patients are doing their routine activities and some are returning to work, they continue to experience pain; however, the pain is at a tolerable level.

Latter part of week one after surgery:

Pain that is experienced during the latter part of the first postsurgical week is usually present during changes of positions such as getting out of bed, standing from a sitting position, or sitting from a standing position. During this time, patients are pain-free while lying down, sitting in a chair, or walking. It is during changes of position, which involves the use of multiple muscles and involvement of the surgical area, that causes the pain to return. In this instance, the pain usually lasts for a few seconds or up to a minute. Once the change in position is completed and the patient is standing, sitting, or walking, they generally have less or no pain at all.

Week two after surgery:

By the second week the pain is described more or less as an "ache." This is a minimal pain which allows complete freedom of movement, but at the same time the patient is made aware that they have had a recent surgery due to this intermittent ache. The ache does not require pain medication and it is not enough to prevent patients from doing their normal work activities. However, the discomfort may *slow down* their abilities. For example, after an eight hour day, patients may only have completed 75% to 85% of their usual workload.

Week three after surgery:

By the third postoperative week most patients will tell me that the pain occasionally "annoys" them. There may be a periodic twinge to remind them that they have had surgery, but it does not substantially slow down their movement. Their flexibility has returned, but they do feel this "pinching" reminder, or an occasional "burning" or "uncomfortable feeling." Once again, this pain does not require any treatment, nor does it diminish the person's ability to resume their regular activities.

Two months after surgery:

By the second month following surgery, patients will have very intermittent pain—for example, pain occurring once a day or once every 2 to 3 days. This will be a minimal to moderate pain that occasionally will stop them in their tracks or "grip" them. This type of a pain tends to return with sudden movements that are unexpected, such as an outburst of laughter, sneezing, or coughing. The pain described does not require treatment; it is merely a reminder of the hernia operation. Patients at this stage have long returned to their work activities. In terms of their ability to return to their recreational activities, they are able to do so with full freedom. However they will find themselves at about 75% to 85% of their pre-injury state.

Six months to one year after surgery:

Moments of pain after hernia surgery may last between six months to one year. During this six month to one year time period the factors involved in pain measurements, such as the intensity, the duration, and the frequency, gradually diminish. The intensity of pain, which is a measure of severity, will diminish to a minimal pain or a "one" on a scale of 0 to 10 with 10 being the severest.

The frequency will also diminish over the first year from every two weeks to about once every six weeks as time progresses.

Additionally, as the pain returns during initiating activities, the amount of time the pain lasts will also diminish. Initially, in the first few days postoperatively the pain would last for ten to thirty minutes—whereas in the post operational six month period, the pain tends to be much smaller and might last 5 to 15 seconds.

I encourage my patients to work through these painful periods. Usually, with progressive time, the pain will diminish to the point where it will be of no consequence to the patient, and will not affect their ability to have normal daily activities and a return to a pre-injury, virtually pain-free state.

CHAPTER EIGHT

Sports Hernias and Abdominal Wall Muscle Strains

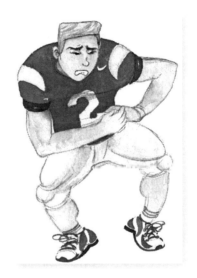

Sports Hernia

A sport hernia is named as such because it typically occurs in professional-level athletes. The hernia is a result of performing activities that are above and beyond what is done (or can be done) by most people. It is highly unusual for a non athlete to develop a sports hernia. A patient who feels that he or she has a sports hernia, and is not playing sports at or near a professional level, is most likely suffering from a muscle strain rather than a sports hernia. Sports hernias affect the groin or inguinal regions much the same as an inguinal or femoral hernia does. The sports hernia is a tear in the muscle tissues without the presence of a hernia sac or bulge. When a sports hernia is present, the abdominal muscles of the athlete are pinching the abdominal contents during particular strenuous activity. This occurs through a slightly enlarged internal inguinal ring or hernia opening.

Diagnosis of a Sports Hernia

The diagnosis of a sports hernia is based on the patient's history and not on physical signs. A sports hernia is a non palpable bulge occurring during strenuous activities typically present in extremely well developed athletes. This occurs when the athlete performs demanding physical activities that would be considered above and beyond what the average individual can perform.

The distinction of a sports hernia from a non sports hernia is based on physical and radiological exam. The distinction factor between a sports hernia and an inguinal hernia occurs in the diagnosis. Inguinal hernias are diagnosed by a physician who determines that a bulge is present. In the absence of a palpable bulge on a physical exam, an inguinal hernia can be seen with the assistance of a radiological exam such as an ultrasound, CT scan, or MRI of the effected part of the body.

Patients with a sports hernia do not have a bulge on physical or radiological examination.

Causes of a Sports Hernia

Sports hernias are caused by strenuous activities of athletes while performing their sport or while training. These sports activities causing the pain are very strenuous events such as the slamming motion of a tennis racket during a serve, running with quick, short cuts while playing football, and extra lifting effort exerted at the very end of weightlifting activity. On occasion, the internal opening of the inguinal canal can be palpable and felt to be larger than normal size, although there is no bulge present. If a palpable bulge is present then the diagnosis would be an inguinal hernia rather than a sports hernia. From the physician's standpoint, the absence of a bulge rules out an inguinal hernia.

Symptoms of a Sports Hernia

The patient who suffers from sports hernia typically has no complaints except for pain at the height of physical activity. For example, they will feel no pain with normal running. But with short turns, or strong speed work, they will complain of a pinching pain in the groin. This occurs because strenuous muscle activities contract their muscles, taxing their body to the point where even a slightly enlarged hernia orifice allows the exit of a small amount of tissue which during the activity becomes pinched. The pinching will cause the athlete to suffer from pain. Since non athletes do not have as well developed muscles as the professional athletes it is unlikely that they will develop a sports hernia.

Physical Signs of a Sports Hernia

Demonstrable physical signs of a hernia are absent. Patients with a sports hernia *do not* have the bulge of a hernia present on radiological exam. The sports hernia is diagnosed based on symptoms alone.

Treatment of a Sports Hernia

Treatment of a sports hernia is essentially the same as that of an inguinal hernia. Without surgery the hernia will not go away. However if the athlete does not perform the particular activity and decides to change to a different, less physically taxing sport, they will not require surgery. For example, I have some elderly patients who are weightlifters. They would rather give up weightlifting than to have surgery. Other patients have told me that they were willing to give up sprinting, and would rather enjoy long and non strenuous running. In other words, if the activity that exacerbates the hernia is stopped, the athlete will not need to have the sports hernia surgery. However, it is advisable to have periodic physical exams, and if it develops into a palpable hernia, surgery will then be required. Whereas, if the pain resolves, there is no further treatment necessary.

Athletes will require surgery to repair the sports hernia if the hernia diminishes their performance. The surgery can be performed using the tension-free mesh technique or the laparoscopic technique. I prefer the open tension-free mesh technique. This technique is normally performed under local anesthesia with sedation but it may be performed under local anesthesia only, or under general anesthesia.

I prefer to perform sports hernia surgery under local anesthesia with sedation because it allows me to test the repair by having the patient strain during surgery. I can then test the integrity of the operation prior to its completion.

This method is done is as follows:

The patient undergoes surgery under deep sedation with a local anesthetic, and after I have placed the mesh, the anesthesiologist arouses the patient. This is done in coordination with the surgeon and the anesthesiologist. I request that they diminish the amount of sedation given to the patient so that they can be aroused. They are still medicated for pain. During this point in the operation, the patient is asked to cough or strain by bearing down. While this is occurring, I examine the operative field for adequate mesh placement. In this manner I am able to perfectly give the patient an exact mesh fit. It is important that I make sure the internal inguinal opening through which the spermaticord exits is neither too loose so that a hernia might reoccur, or too tight thereby causing a painful spermaticord. Thus, by performing the surgery under local anesthesia with sedation, the exact fit can be securely accomplished. This ensures that the patient will get the best possible surgical result with the strongest repair and least postoperative pain, and lessening the amount of recovery time. This will enable the athlete to return to their sports activities with minimal down time.

Abdominal Wall Muscle Strain

An abdominal wall strain is an injury that can occur to any portion of the abdominal wall where there is muscle tissue. The abdominal wall strain may affect any of the muscles including the muscles of the groin. When this occurs, it is commonly known as a groin strain or a pulled groin muscle. The muscles of the abdomen are strained typically during strenuous activities whereby the muscles become pulled due to lifting, pushing, or pulling forces. Any one of these forces can cause the muscles to tear.

When the muscle is torn, there is a small amount of bleeding. This may result in swelling, and/or commonly severe pain in the effected muscle. This painful area may at times be confused with the presence of a hernia. A muscle strain is not a hernia. A muscle strain can however develop into a hernia. If a weakened, strained muscle does not completely heal, it may further tear resulting in a hernia. Typically, the muscle strain occurs in areas where hernias frequent, such as the umbilical region and the groin.

The symptoms of a muscle strain typically are unrelenting pain in the site of the strain with movement or change in position. As the muscles are being stretched, the pain is increased. This occurs due to the injured muscles causing an irritation of nerves in and around the muscle tissue. Patients suffering from a muscle strain complain of pain with movement and especially with lifting. With increasingly heavy lifting the pain increases.

The main difference between a strain and a hernia is that severe pain is more common with a strain than with hernias. The hernia pain typically occurs with heavy lifting only. The pain associated with a muscle strain also occurs with either movement or position change.

In the early stages of hernia development however, the pain of the hernia is similar to that of a strain. The pain associated with an early hernia usually resolves within the week. When the pain resolves there may be a bulge present. The pain with a muscle strain usually resolves within 2 to 6 weeks. During the resolution period, patients typically complain that although the pain has not completely gone away, it has diminished in intensity over time. A patient who has a muscle pain for a period of 4 to 6 weeks will generally state that although the pain is still bothersome, on a relative scale the pain is considerably less than what it was, as compared to the initial phase.

Although the pain associated with a muscle strain is typically located at the site of the pulled muscle, the pain may also radiate since the nerves travel along a path particular for the nerve. The pain then radiates along the path of these nerves. Therefore, the pain of a muscle strain affecting the abdominal muscles may radiate around the flank. A strain affecting the groin muscles may radiate to the scrotal area, as well as the upper thigh regions, and to the back. On examination, the area that is affected by the strain might be slightly swollen or very tender. This may be distinguished from a hernia that is typically non tender except for the very early acute phases. Tenderness usually involves irritation of the nerve as a result of intra muscular bleeding from the strain.

Treatment of an Abdominal Wall Strain

The treatment for an abdominal strain is resting the effected muscle. Initially strains are treated with a 1 to 2 day period of placing cold (ice pack) to the area. In the initial stages the application of cold is used to diminish the blood supply to the area and thereby reduce swelling. After a couple days muscle strains are treated with a heat compress. Applying heat at this period will increase the circulation to the affected area, assisting the removal of toxins and blood clots.

Usually over-the-counter medications will suffice for pain relief. At times, prescription medication may be needed for severe cases of abdominal wall strains. It is advised that patients diminish or stop strenuous activities. By following these steps, a strain will usually heal in 10 days to 2 weeks. However, in the case of professional athletes, frequently they are unable to stop their work because of the team's schedule, and by continuing to work they are perpetuating the strain itself. Therefore, the strain, rather than healing in a couple weeks, may last for a prolonged period of time; perhaps as long as up to 6 months.

If you do not rest an abdominal muscle strain, the strain may become chronic, lasting for several months. In any event, given sufficient time, an abdominal wall strain will eventually completely heal on its own without surgery.

CHAPTER NINE

Complications of Hernias

Complications may occur after any operation. Typically your surgeon will discuss with you the most common possible complications of your operation. They will not usually discuss the less common complications unless you request them to do so. The least common complications are those that occur in less than 0.2 percent of the patients, or one out of 500 patients.

I will begin this chapter by mentioning the lesser common complications of hernia surgery. These complications are not unique to hernias, and may occur after *any* operation. The least common and most severe complication of any surgery, of course, is death, and when this results, more often than not it is from an adverse or unexpected reaction to anesthesia. The death rate is about 5 to 6 out of a million. I tell my patients that the risk of driving home from surgery is greater than the risk of the operation. Other risks include myocardial infarction or heart attack, or pulmonary embolism. Patients with preexisting heart disease, or obesity, are at a greater risk of developing these complications.

An allergic reaction affects five percent of patients. The most common allergic reaction is a rash. The lesser common reactions are hives, causing difficulty breathing, and in extremely rare cases even death. Although not considered an allergic reaction, some patients have drug sensitivities and develop nausea and vomiting. This is commonly caused by pain medications that contain codeine or one of its derivatives—or anti-inflammatory non steriodals such as Motrin and Advil.

Swelling, or a hematoma, frequently occurs after surgery. But this is not considered a complication unless the postoperative bleeding is severe. The lesser forms of postoperative swelling results in a purplish discoloration of the genitalia, and this affects as much as 10 percent of the patients.

All patients have pain after hernia surgery. In a few cases, the pain can last for several months. Pain is not considered a complication unless it either remains severe for months after surgery, or becomes chronic. Chronic pain may be mild and/or severe, but remains up to one year after surgery. Chronic pain affects only 3 to 5 percent of all hernia patients.

The complications of hernia surgery that are unique to hernia operations include chronic pain, bleeding, infection, and hernia recurrence. Bleeding may occur in less than 1 percent of the patients, and only about one in a thousand require a procedure to stop the bleeding.

Infections occur in about 1 to 2 percent of the patients, and are most frequently treated with antibiotic ointment. Occasionally, patients require a course of antibiotics. An infection requiring the removal of mesh is very rare. I have never had to remove an infected mesh in any patient that I have operated on.

The recurrence rate for a first time hernia repair is 0.5 percent. My personal recurrence rate is 0.2 percent.

Possible Inguinal Hernia Surgery Complications

Based on the national average these are the complications following a routine inguinal hernia surgery on a healthy individual. They are as follows:

- Recurrence of hernia: 0.5% or 1 in 200.
- Infection of the incision: 0.5% or 1 in 200.

- Bleeding after surgery: 1% or 1 in 100.

- Change in testicular size or function: 1% or 1 in 100.

- Injury to the bladder or bowel: 0.025% or 1 in 400.

- Injury to the vas deferens: 0.025% or 1 in 400.

- Temporary incisional pain lasting 2 to 3 months: 3 to 5% or 3 to 5 in 100.

- Mild chronic incisional pain with neuroma formation that is non debilitating: 1% or 1 in 100.

- Chronic incisional pain with neuroma formation that is debilitating: 0.5% or 1 in 200.

- Temporary swelling or black and blue in the region of the surgery lasting one week: 10% or 1 in 10. [Note: The temporary swelling or black and blueness are not considered a complication.]

The majority of patients will have numbness in the area surrounding the surgery. As the nerves regenerate from the periphery of the incision, sensation slowly returns to the area. Eventually the area of permanent numbness beneath the incision will diminish to a small region approximately the size of a quarter. The numbness is barely noticeable to most patients and does not alter any normal function. The permanent numbness is the result of cutting superficial nerves in the skin. This numbness is not considered a complication, rather it is routine and present in all postoperative patients.

The complications postoperatively are increased in certain individuals. The above statistics do not apply for these individuals. There are a larger number of complications in patients who have recurrent hernias, obese patients, patients that are immune compromised, elderly patients, patients with infections when the surgery is done on an emergency basis, and on patients with strangulated hernias.

Post Operative Neuroma

I had the following conversation with a male patient who came to me after having hernia surgery performed by another surgeon. He was frustrated and complaining of chronic pain which had failed to resolve after conservative treatment.

Dr. Albin: Essentially what has happened to you is that you've had the surgery and more than likely you are having pain as the result of an injury to one or more nerves that are in the area of the groin. This is called a nerve injury, or neuroma. This is when the nerves have actually been damaged by the surgery. Sometimes it is the result of cutting the nerves, and sometimes pain occurs when the mesh becomes stuck to the nerves. In any event, the appropriate treatment has already been done by your doctor at this point. You have already received pain medications and injections without relief.

You are going to have to consider continuing to take the medication and the treatment that is being done by the pain management specialist. Alternatively, what I'm doing is explaining to you the next step which would be to consider surgery. Now, the reason why they have not offered you surgery as a sooner step is because the results of neuroma surgery are not that great. It's not like hernia surgery where you simply have a common hernia repaired—the doctor fixes the hernia and you're done. You have a hernia surgery complication, and the complication is nerve injury.

I can offer a surgery that will possibly correct the problem. The reason why I say "possibly" is because the correction result is not a guarantee. Up to this point none of your doctors have offered you neuroma surgery because there is no easy way to fix a neuroma, even with an operation. The operation that I perform involves reopening and exploring the previous surgery—looking around and identifying the nerves that have been affected in the region. I would actually cut the ends of the nerves and bury them in the muscle so that they would become less sensitive. At the same time, I would look at the mesh. If the mesh is too tight, or trapping the spermaticord, I would free it up and make sure it's not at all tight. When the mesh is too tight, it can also pinch a nerve.

This is essentially the operation. It is a lengthy operation. It can take approximately two hours. However, the results are not as successful as a hernia operation. The results we expect are that 40 percent of our patients will be completely cured of the pain. When I say cured, I mean 90 to 95 percent very satisfied. There are about 40 percent of the people who will not be cured, but will still be better off. For example, moderate pain may become minimal pain. This is not quite the same as making the pain go away, but not as bad as the pain initially was. One major problem with this operation is that there is a 15 percent chance where there may be no change. These patients come back and say, "I feel the same—this has been a complete waste of my time." And I would be remiss if I did not warn you that there is a 5 percent chance where patients may actually get worse. This occurs when there is severe scarring, and I have to go in and clean up. Sometimes I may inadvertently cut other nerves.

So to be frank, no other surgeon has offered you neuroma surgery because the results are considered poor. It is not a good choice. But presently it is the only alternative you have if you are suffering from severe pain that has not diminished with conservative treatment.

Patient: *Why is it possible that I am still going to have a problem if you are going to cut the nerves?*

Dr. Albin: Nerves have a memory. In addition, they are like two stranded electrical cords. There is a current going to the body telling you to move your legs, and a current coming back and telling you that you are feeling pain. Certain patients feel pain after the nerves have been cut. For example, some patients who have had a leg amputation can feel as if they are wiggling their toes because their nerves are sending a message back saying that the toes are wiggling. This is the memory of the nerves. This is the basis behind patients feeling continuous pain even after undergoing neuroma surgery. It is the reason that neuroma surgery is not always successful. And as I said, this is the reason why many surgeons do not perform this surgery.

Patient: *How long will my recovery period be?*

Dr. Albin: The recovery for neuroma surgery is similar to that of hernia surgery, four to six weeks.

Patient: *I feel I have no choice, Doctor Albin, I'm tired of having this pain and if this operation can help me, I want to try.*

Dr. Albin: Are you working now?

Patient: *No I am disabled.*

Dr. Albin: And is this pain the only reason for your disability?

Patient: *No, I have many reasons for disability, including a heart problem. But if you cure me of this pain, I will be less disabled. I am willing to go ahead with this operation if I have at least a forty percent chance that my pain will be cured.*

Since that patient had severe disabling cardiac problems, in my opinion, I felt that the risk of a lengthy surgery could result in him having a heart attack, and even death. On my recommendation, the patient consulted his cardiologist and together they decided that the operation was too risky. Ultimately the patient was able to modify his lifestyle and was able to cope with his pain.

An Athlete's Post Surgical Questions

I had the following conversation with a female athlete who, after having hernia surgery by another surgeon, was having pain four weeks postoperatively. She came to me for a second opinion after the postoperative visit with her surgeon seemed to be rushed and short on reassuring information.

Patient: *I am a volleyball athlete. I had a "mesh inguinal hernia repair" four weeks ago and my doctor returned me to all activities "within tolerance." I continue to have pain in my groin during practices. I play collegiate volleyball and I am in our preseason phase, six hours of practice a day, in two practice sessions. I have stopped weightlifting at this time. How do I continue to practice without causing big problems for myself?*

Dr. Albin: You may be healing slowly from your surgery, or you may have reinjured yourself by straining a muscle. You may have to ease into your practice. It may take two to four weeks to get to six hours of practice per day. Ice up the surgical site after each practice. If the pain accelerates after a practice, you may have to sit out for a day or two. As a general rule, if it hurts, do not do it.

For the time being, back off on exercises that accelerate the groin pain. Apply warm compresses to the area, or just sit in a hot tub daily several times a day. Take over-the-counter non steroidal analgesics such as Motrin, Advil, or Aleve. If this does not resolve your pain, then consider an evaluation for surgery.

The patient followed my recommendations, and fortunately surgery was not necessary, and she only had to sit out the opening week of her volleyball season.

Hernia Specialists Have Fewer Complications

General surgery is a vast field encompassing many body systems. It is difficult to be an expert in everything. I decided to become an expert in only one portion of general surgery. This is why I became a hernia specialist.

As a hernia specialist I pride myself in having such a low complication rate. I have never had a hernia patient die. I operate on a large number of patients. Some weeks I perform twenty-five hernia operations in a week. I cannot afford to take chances with my patients. I have to give them the best operation possible. Many of my patients come to me as a referral from another surgeon. Many of my patients travel to see me from all over the United States and throughout the world.

My complication rate is well below the average. I take the time to perform each and every operation carefully. I have a surgical crew that has been with me for several years. We have performed thousands of hernia operations together. We are meticulous when it comes to sterility in the operating room. I have much less infections than in the hospital. Of course, that is to be expected because there are a lot of sick patients, and even some sick working personnel in the hospitals. I am never rushed. I identify the patient's anatomy prior to performing my hernia repair. My patients get a hernia repair that is customized to fit their individual needs. Some of my patients tell me that they expected that they would have more discomfort after surgery. Many of my patients congratulate me during their first postoperative visit for a job well done.

The good news is that I am not alone in my conscientiousness. There are plenty of very good hernia surgeons out there. So use due diligence: do your research, which includes seeking referrals from other medical professionals (such as urologists and gynecologists); plus getting recommendations from other satisfied hernia surgery patients. Make the effort and you will be able to find a hernia surgeon you can absolutely count on to do your operation right the first time.

AFTERWORD

Even a Hernia Specialist Can Get a Hernia

Anyone can develop a hernia. And like the chapter title says, "Even a *hernia specialist* can get a hernia." No one is immune, including me. Still, can you imagine my surprise? Here I know everything there is to know about hernia prevention, and yet I also personally developed an inguinal hernia and had to have hernia surgery

One of the reasons I wrote this book was to help those people (and there are a surprising number of them) who are embarrassed about having a hernia. These patients are often athletes who are in top shape. They always thought it was the out-of-shape people, with weak stomach muscles, who got hernias. As a specialist, I know better. I know that no one is exempt. But the most embarrassing part for me was that I developed my hernia while writing this book. I suppose some of my colleagues are having a pretty good laugh on that one.

But let them laugh, because the way I see it, every experience in life, no matter how bad it may seem at the time, has an upside. In this case, having a hernia has made me a better hernia doctor. Think about it...how many doctors have you been to who are diagnosing a condition they've never themselves had? For example, most cardiologists have never had a heart attack. And most oncologists have never had cancer. Thus, they don't know what it truly *feels* like to be a patient with the condition they are diagnosing and prescribing treatment for.

I can now say to every one of my patients, "I know what you are going through!" And I can say it with heartfelt conviction. How many times have you heard a medical professional calmly say, "I know what you must be feeling?" And you wanted to shout back, "NO YOU DON'T!"

Well, that will never happen with me. I now know exactly what my patients are going through, and here's why...

In my off time, when I'm not practicing medicine, I am a triathlete. I have been participating in triathlon races for the past eight years. Triathlon races involve three sports: swimming, biking, and running. During my first year as a triathlete I participated in a total of 10 sprint triathlons. This is a short race which usually lasts no longer than one and a half hours. During my second year I moved up in distance to the half Ironman category when I completed the Wildflower Triathlon for the first time. The Wildflower Half Ironman Triathlon race is a longer distance. It consists of a 1.2 mile swim, 56 miles on a bike, and a 13.1 mile run. I completed my first full Ironman race during my third year as a triathlete. The Ironman race consists of a 2.4 mile swim, a 112 mile bike, and a 26.2 mile marathon run. It took me 14 hours and 26 minutes to complete the race. Presently, each year I usually participate in at least one Ironman race, one Half Ironman Race, and several sprint triathlons.

I generally begin training about six months in advance of my races. Just two weeks prior to a scheduled Half Ironman race, the Wildflower Triathlon, I was diagnosed with an inguinal hernia. This particular race is known to be the third most difficult Ironman race due to it being a hilly race, so I was faced with a tough decision.

As a hernia specialist and triathlete I have always been very careful in trying to prevent myself from developing a hernia. I am very aware of the do's and don'ts with regard to lifting and straining. I follow the proper techniques during my exercise routines. Even though I possess this knowledge I still was unable to prevent myself from developing an inguinal hernia.

I believe that no one activity caused my hernia, rather my hernia developed as a result of performing strenuous activities over a period of several years. However, I feel the main culprit was biking in the hills and mountains of Southern California. Triathletes tend to work out to the point where they experience what we refer to as "tolerable pain." As a result, triathletes are known to have a high threshold for pain. While training for a race I bike 200 to 250 miles each week. In order to increase my strength on the bike, I bike on hills. The amount of power needed to bike up a steep hill is similar to pushing heavy weights with your legs in the gym, called the leg press. The main difference between biking up a steep hill and pushing leg weights is that the gym workout is more strenuous, but the uphill bike ride lasts for a longer period of time. I have climbed our local mountain, Mount Wilson, which consists of a 5000 foot climb over 18 miles, numerous times as a training ride. It is my opinion that the strenuous nature of spending hours on a bike climbing steep hills each week had weakened my abdominal wall muscles and resulted in the hernia.

While I was on a six mile training run for the Wildflower Triathlon, I felt something funny in my left groin area. I pushed on a squishy bump and heard a gurgling sound. I had just discovered my own left inguinal hernia. I was shocked to discover that not only did I have a hernia, but that I was going to need surgery—and soon. My first reaction was, "This cannot be happening to me!" My second reaction was, "What am I going to tell my wife and family and friends?" I then finished up my run at a slightly slower pace.

I then had to decide whether I was well enough to race at Wildflower, or whether I should throw in the towel and have surgery immediately. My race was exactly two weeks away.

At this time in my training, my workouts consisted of about two workouts a day, six days a week, with one day of rest. My workouts included three days of running, three days of biking, three days of swimming, and two days of weightlifting. I decided that I would give up the weightlifting for now.

I soon discovered that swimming had no effect on my hernia. I also discovered that biking had no effect except for very steep hills. I remembered that the Wildflower Triathlon has one steep hill which is called "Nasty Grade" due to a precipitous 900 foot climb. But the hernia had no effect on my bike *speed* workouts, so I could continue with them.

Running, however, was a problem. I found I could run up to six miles pain free. As a result of being in the upright position, running became problematic after six miles when my hernia began to protrude. I was comfortable running the flats, but not the hills. So I ran the flats and walked the hills. The last week, even running flats became painful, so I had to stop running.

I spoke to my coach and we put together a race plan based on my hernia. It was obviously quite different from a non hernia race plan. Most importantly, I made a commitment to myself to let the hernia be my guide. Were it to become too painful, I would then and there quit the race. I also decided that I would avoid looking at my watch or my heart rate except at the end of each of the three events: swim, bike, and run. I wanted to race by "feel" — except on the bike, during which time I would use a wattage meter and race at my pre-designated level of 140 watts.

Wildflower Triathlon, Lake San Antonio, California...

At 9:05 the gun went off for my wave of the race.

I ran into the water from the swim starting line. There was the usual pushing and kicking during the first 200M of the swim course as the athletes are bunched up in a tightly knit group. After the 200M buoy, I quickly got into my usual swim form. Before long I was at the swim turn around. Then there was the sprint back to the shore. I completed the 1.2 mile swim in 39:22 minutes (1:50 / 100 yards), a personal record for that race. I was in the top 50 percentile in my age group for the swim.

I quickly removed my swim gear and changed into my bike gear. Within a few minutes I was on the bike. The hernia never bothered me while I rode the bike except for the very steep hills. I biked hard and fast but kept to my 140 watt fitness level. I was feeling good and kept up with my training level for the first 40 miles. Mile 41 is where Nasty Grade begins and it never felt this hard to me before. I persisted and kept in form as I biked this steep incline. Luckily the hernia never bothered me. I finished the 56 mile bike ride in 3 hours 43 minutes 48 seconds (15 miles/hour) a personal best for me for that race. I was also in the top 50 percentile in my age group for the bike ride.

I was staring the 13.1 mile run feeling tired. It was 81 degrees and I had been racing about four and a half hours. I decided to continue with my race plan, which was to stay in my comfort level. I ran the flat and downhill portions of the race. But I walked the uphill. I felt fine for the first nine miles. The last two miles were uncomfortable and painful. I continued at a steady pace to run the last two miles of flats and walk the hills. I finished at a pretty good time considering that I was injured. My overall time was 7 hours 13 minutes. I placed 27th of 46 in my age group. I had finished the race very close to the average time for my age group, and what is considered a good competitive time.

Three days after the race I had one of my colleagues at the Hernia Center of Southern California repair my left inguinal hernia.

Here's what I learned firsthand: It is possible to train and exercise with a hernia; but you will perform at suboptimal levels. It is obviously better to be healthy and fit and train at your optimal fitness level.

I also learned that we must prepare ourselves for whatever life has to offer. My advice to my family, friends and patients is that it is important to remain healthy. First and foremost, if we are healthy, we will feel good about ourselves and gain self-confidence to pursue the challenges that life has to offer. Staying fit gives us the energy we need to help ourselves and others. We must put in the time and effort by training hard in order to stay healthy and fit. When you have a healthy mind and a healthy body, life is beautiful and you can enjoy all that it has to offer.

When you wake up each morning say to yourself:
- I will maintain my health at the highest possible level.
- I will stay fit by maintaining a daily or weekly workout routine.
- I will work out or train hard, but safely.
- I will work out or race at my fitness level.
- Today is my day—I will enjoy my life.

THE ALBIN TECHNIQUE

A New, Revolutionary Method for Hernia Repair

I discovered my new technique by combining several other well-established surgical techniques. My new technique is a variation of the standard technique for hernia repair. Most surgeons follow proven surgical principles and vary their technique. After reviewing multiple surgical techniques, I evaluated the advantages and disadvantages of each one, and was able to devise a technique that puts into one operation the best of each method. Thus, the new *Albin Technique* is the only one I now perform for inguinal hernias.

For the past year my groundbreaking inguinal hernia technique has been very successful on the first 500 patients. The preliminary results are extraordinary and have been very predictable. My postoperative patients have minimal postoperative complaints. I have not had a single recurrence with this with this technique after the first 500 patients. There is a high satisfaction rate with early return to work and activities, and minimal patient complaints.

As of this writing, I am in the process of preparing a paper regarding The Albin Technique for publication in medical and surgical journals, as well as a presentation at the Hernia Society meeting.

The Albin Technique utilizes a non absorbable polypropylene mesh and a combination of absorbable and permanent sutures. The advantage of this technique is that it is devised to better repair as well as to prevent additional hernias from occurring in other adjacent locations.

The new technique places the mesh in-between the muscles layers of the abdominal wall. Tissue trauma is minimized by not placing the mesh behind the muscles as is done in some standard methods. The mesh and the muscles scar together in-between the layers of the muscle resulting in a stronger hernia repair. The mesh used is large enough to blanket the floor of the inguinal canal and surrounding muscles preventing another hernia from occurring.

The mesh is sutured in place using a permanent suture in the inner or medial aspect of the inguinal floor. On the outer or lateral aspect, an absorbable suture is utilized because this is the portion of the inguinal canal that is most prone to a nerve injury. Unlike the permanent sutures that are commonly used, the absorbable sutures dissolve so that permanent nerve injury will not likely occur. This additionally facilitates nerve healing. The mesh is sutured together around the lower portion of the spermaticord. This technique minimizes pressure on the spermaticord resulting in a significant decrease in pain and damage to the testicle. In regard to females, there is minimal disturbance of the round ligament of the uterus resulting also in a satisfactory result.

My technique differs from standard hernia repairs in the following ways:
- I use a larger mesh to prevent additional hernias from occurring in other locations on the same side as the hernia.
- I use absorbable sutures in the region of the nerves to prevent permanent nerve injuries.
- My mesh is sutured in place below the spermaticord to minimize testicular injury.

- The operation is equally beneficial to both man and women.

Results:

- Since developing this technique one year ago, I have not had a single hernia recurrence on the same side.
- My patients have a significant decrease in postoperative pain.
- They use less pain pills and,
- Return to work sooner.
- My patients also return to sports and other recreational activities sooner.
- Since my operation both is designed to provide an immediate repair of the hernia and the prevention of a recurrent hernia in the same side, my patients return to both work and exercise one week after surgery. Imagine a safe hernia operation with only one week down time!
- When my patients see me in my office after the operation during their postoperative visits, I know they are pleased with the results by the smiles on their faces. They often shake my hand and tell me that they are glad they chose to go with the new technique.

For more information on The Albin Technique, call (626) 584-6116 or e-mail to dralbin@earthlink.net

ABOUT THE AUTHOR

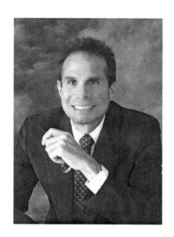

Dr. David Albin is the Medical Director for the Hernia Center of Southern California and the Pasadena Surgery Center, LLC. A recognized expert in hernia repair, Dr. Albin has performed over 8000 hernia surgeries. Certified by the American Board of General Surgery, a fellow of the American College of Surgeons and a Qualified Medical Examiner, Dr. Albin has authored many published medical articles and has been appointed to the staff of several respected hospitals.

He graduated from Kasturba Medical School and then went on to attend a one year clerkship at Buffalo Medical School in New York. Dr. Albin completed his internship at the Downstate Medical Center before moving to California and completing his residency in surgery at King/Drew UCLA Medical Center.

Dr. Albin started his general surgical practice in Los Angeles, California in 1987. As a highly qualified trauma surgeon he remained affiliated with the King/Drew UCLA Medical Center where he worked for several years as a trauma team leader in the general surgical residency program trauma center where he was able to teach other surgeons the principles of surgery.

Dr. Albin, determined to refine his surgical techniques, became sub-specialized in the field of herniology. It is easy to know a little about a lot of things but to know everything is almost impossible. It was this ideology that brought Dr. Albin in to his present field as one of the few experts in herniology, or hernia repair. This field is small enough that you can know it all and know it perfectly and Dr. Albin feels he has accomplished this, which is why he now devotes his entire surgical practice to hernia repair, and has even perfected his own hernia surgical procedure, "The Albin Technique". Dr. Albin feels it is important to remain abreast with the recent changes in the field of hernia repair. He attends the national and international hernia surgical meetings and reviews all of the journals as a means of staying informed with the advancements in this sub-specialty. He is a teacher, author, and medical legal expert in the field of hernia repair. Dr. Albin is known throughout Los Angeles County as the surgeon to see for hernias. He is the hernia surgeon for the Los Angeles Police Department, Sheriff Department, California Highway Patrol, Los Angeles City and County Fire Departments and the Los Angeles Unified School District. In addition to many athletes, hernia patents from throughout the United States and the world come to Dr. Albin for hernia surgery.

Dr. Albin believes in the importance of fitness. He is an accomplished triathlete and has completed five Ironman events; the Ironman New Zealand 2008, Ironman Switzerland 2007, Ironman Florida 2006, Ironman Malaysia 2006, and the Ironman Coeur D'Alene in Idaho 2005. He has also completed in six Half Ironman triathlons at Wildflower, Half Vineman, and the California Half Ironman. Dr. Albin believes in putting his own advice into practice, which is how he has been able to continually place in the top of his age group in Sprint and Olympic distance triathlon events. He placed second in his age group in the Los Angeles Triathlon in 2007.

Dr. Albin is married and his wife is a physician practicing obstetrics and gynecology. He is the proud father of four children, all of whom are triathletes. His youngest son, Ben, placed first in his age group in the 2005 Los Angeles Triathlon. His oldest son Dr. Michael Albin is attending a general surgical residency at North Shore Hospital in New York.

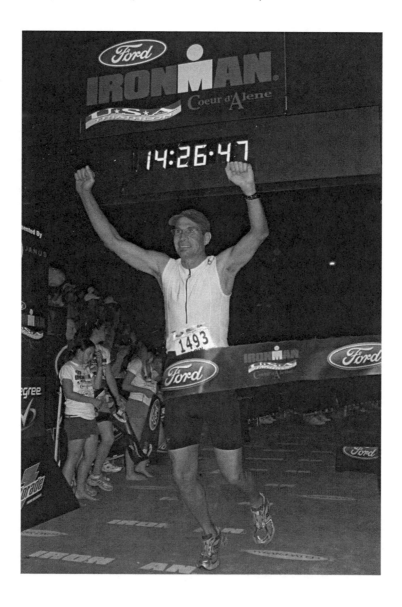

INDEX

T
tennis, 86–87
tension-free mesh technique, 10–11, 35, 43–46, 58–59, 60
tests for diagnosis, 28, 49
travel, 72

U
ultrasound, 49
umbilical hernias
    congenital, 64–65
    cosmetic concerns, 67–69
    described, 32–33, 63–65
    key-hole surgery, 68–69
    recurrence, 68
    treatment of, 66–67
urinary symptoms, 26–27
urological dysfunction, 11

V
ventral hernias, 38–40
vomiting, 26

W
website, 2
weightlifting, 42–43, 84–85
women
    cosmetic concerns, 67–69
    groin hernias, 6–7
    pregnant, 9
work, returning to, 14, 77–80
wound care, 76

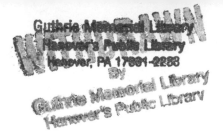
CPSIA information can be obtained at www.ICGtesting.com
Printed in the USA
LVOW062043231211

260882LV00002B/223/P